Caregiver's Guide

MCFARLAND HEALTH TOPICS SERIES

Living with Multiple Chemical Sensitivity: Narratives of Coping.
Gail McCormick. 2001

Graves' Disease: A Practical Guide.
Elaine A. Moore with Lisa Moore. 2001

Autoimmune Diseases and Their Environmental Triggers.
Elaine A. Moore. 2002

Hepatitis: Causes, Treatments and Resources.
Elaine A. Moore. 2006

Arthritis: A Patient's Guide.
Sharon E. Hohler, RN. 2008

The Promise of Low Dose Naltrexone Therapy: Potential Benefits in Cancer, Autoimmune, Neurological and Infectious Disorders.
Elaine A. Moore and Samantha Wilkinson. 2009

Living with HIV: A Patient's Guide.
Mark Cichocki, RN. 2009

Understanding Multiple Chemical Sensitivity: Causes, Effects, Personal Experiences and Resources.
Els Valkenburg. 2010

Type 2 Diabetes: Social and Scientific Origins, Medical Complications and Implications for Patients and Others.
Andrew Kagan, M.D. 2010

The Amphetamine Debate: The Use of Adderall, Ritalin and Related Drugs for Behavior Modification, Neuroenhancement and Anti-Aging Purposes.
Elaine A. Moore. 2011

CCSVI as the Cause of Multiple Sclerosis: The Science Behind the Controversial Theory. Marie A. Rhodes. 2011

Coping with Post-Traumatic Stress Disorder: A Guide for Families, 2d ed. Cheryl A. Roberts. 2011

Living with Insomnia: A Guide to Causes, Effects and Management, with Personal Accounts.
Phyllis L. Brodsky and Allen Brodsky. 2011

Caregiver's Guide
Care for Yourself While You Care for Your Loved Ones

SHARON E. HOHLER

MCFARLAND HEALTH TOPICS SERIES
Elaine A. Moore, *Series Editor*

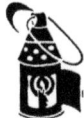

McFarland & Company, Inc., Publishers
Jefferson, North Carolina, and London

Disclaimer: The information presented in this book is for educational purposes and should not be taken as medical advice. Readers are encouraged to seek competent medical care, learn about the resources available and work with their doctors to improve their health status. Advances in medical knowledge and care will render the information in this book (at present accurate and timely) out of date. Individuals are encouraged to use the reputable resources listed to know the latest and best information.

LIBRARY OF CONGRESS CATALOGUING-IN-PUBLICATION DATA

Hohler, Sharon E., 1953–
    Caregiver's guide : care for yourself while you care for your loved ones / Sharon E. Hohler.
      p.   cm. — (McFarland Health Topics)
    Includes bibliographical references and index.

    ISBN 978-0-7864-4962-0
    softcover : acid free paper ∞

    1. Caregivers — Health and hygiene.   I. Title.
RA645.3.H64   2012
362'.0425 — dc23   2011039194

BRITISH LIBRARY CATALOGUING DATA ARE AVAILABLE

© 2012 Sharon E. Hohler. All rights reserved

No part of this book may be reproduced or transmitted in any form or by any means, electronic or mechanical, including photocopying or recording, or by any information storage and retrieval system, without permission in writing from the publisher.

Front cover images © 2012 Shutterstock.com

Manufactured in the United States of America

McFarland & Company, Inc., Publishers
  Box 611, Jefferson, North Carolina 28640
    www.mcfarlandpub.com

To David, thanks for your love and support.
Here is book #2

To my partners in caregiving, thank you. You are the greatest.
This includes my siblings
Dorothy and Peggy and their families
and David's siblings Teresa, Robert, Martha,
Janet, Mark and Joseph and their families.

Table of Contents

Acknowledgments ix
Preface 1

SECTION I. CAREGIVING

1. Statistics and Stages of Caregiving 5
2. Children Involved in Caregiving 21
3. Caregivers Need Care Too 32
4. Stress Breakers 46
5. Looking Back Through History 60
6. All Things Medical 74
7. All Things Surgical 107
8. Practical Decisions 126
9. Grieving and Remembering 141
10. Strategies for Healthy Aging 152

SECTION II. COMMON HEALTH PROBLEMS ENCOUNTERED

11. Alzheimer's Disease 165
12. Arthritis 179
13. Cancer 193

| 14. Diabetes | 207 |
| 15. Heart Disease | 223 |

Glossary	237
Chapter Notes	241
Resources	257
Index	269

Acknowledgments

Thank you to loving family and friends who supported us and listened to us during our caregiving time.

Thank you to my proofreaders, David and Peggy, who took their valuable time to read and improve my manuscript.

Thank you to those who shared their stories in this book: Cindy Brotherton and family; C. Kip Bennett and son; Katie Bond, daughters Jan, Sue and families; Jessica Hill and family; Peggy Gross and family.

Thank you to medical and nursing colleagues who contribute much to my knowledge.

Thank you to friends at Heartland Writers Guild and Missouri Writers Guild who taught me how to be successful at writing.

Preface

Sixty-five million people give care to their frail, ailing, or disabled loved ones every year. My family experienced this phenomenon. My parents died at ages 88 and 92 from heart and cardiovascular disease after several years of declining health. David's mother developed Alzheimer's disease and died at age 85. Our family (both sides) including siblings, and the grandchildren were great partners in helping care for our loved ones. They pulled together and supported us and each other.

For some families, caregiving begins gradually and builds. That was the case in my family. Visiting to socialize became inadequate. Mom and Dad changed from two whole individuals into two halves that barely made a whole.

A grandson began to care for their yard and we daughters began to cook extra food and take lunch. Out-of-town family came for a visit and power-washed the exterior of their house and cut limbs off a tree. We knew we were helping conserve the energy of our parents. As their needs increased, the family tried to fill the gaps. We didn't recognize we had become caregivers until after Mom's death when Dad wanted to finish out his life living at home. He died at age 92 at home.

For other families, a crisis calls for caregiving. When mom falls and breaks her hip, changes (at least temporarily) must be made to care for her while she recuperates.

Many families don't recognize that they have become caregivers. And yet research has shown that people who identify themselves as caregivers fare better. They learn about Dad's health issues and can start to work with his doctor. They learn what resources are available and begin to utilize the help that's available, whether it's family, friends or agencies.

Caregivers must make self-care a priority so that they will have the health and energy to care for their loved one. The alternative is exhaustion and potential burnout. A healthy attitude toward caregiving begins when a person recognizes that (1) he is a caregiver, (2) he cannot do this alone, and (3) he gets organized and utilizes the resources available to him and his family. Throughout this book, the caregiver is admonished to also "care for himself."

How does a caregiver care for herself when up to her elbows with the daily chores of caring for a loved one? Chapter 3, "Caregivers Need Care Too," gives any caregiver the "permission" to care for herself and reasons why she should. Chapter 4, "Stress Breakers," gives a variety of activities which a caregiver can utilize to decrease her own stress. Chapter 10 "Aging Gracefully" provides recommendations from medical experts that a person can use to promote health.

After a person realizes he or she is caregiving, then what happens? Most of the caregiving recipients have health issues. The medical world is complex and confusing. Chapter 6, "All Things Medical," and Chapter 7, "All Things Surgical," strive to simplify and explain the medical world to caregivers. Several valuable documents (from The Joint Commission [JCAHO]) have been included. A caregiver can benefit from information such as "Tips for Your Doctor Visit" and "How to Avoid Mistakes in Your Medicines."

Chapter 8, "Practical Decisions," focuses on safety issues around the home. Is home a safe place for the frail, elderly person to live? The International Association of Certified Home Inspectors provides suggestions on how to make home safer and prevent falls, fires, and carbon monoxide poisoning. When the electricity goes off, what should a caregiving family do to keep their loved ones safe and prevent overheating in summertime and hypothermia in the winter? The American Geriatric Society gives valuable information for these situations.

A painful part of caregiving is grieving the death of loved ones. It's an inevitable part of life and caregiving. Chapter 9, "Grieving and Remembering," recounts one family's experiences as they deal with the loss of their loved one.

The last five chapters give information on five common health problems: Alzheimer's disease, arthritis, cancer, diabetes and heart disease (heart attacks, stroke and congestive heart failure). Each chapter explains what the disease is, who is at risk for developing the disease, whether a person can prevent or delay the development of the disease, an explanation of what happens during the disease, diagnosis and treatments in language that nonmedical people can understand.

The families who shared their stories with the world make this book special. All other names in this book are fictitious names attached to real-life events that happened to our family and friends. We thank them and encourage all caregivers to care for yourself as you care for your loved ones.

SECTION I. CAREGIVING

1

Statistics and Stages of Caregiving

RRRRing.

"Hello?"

"Hi, are you Jon Jones? My name is Bertha Smith and I live in Memphis, Tennessee. Your mama parked her car in front of my house and walked to my door. She said, 'I'm lost, please call my son Jon.' She found your phone number in her purse and asked me to call. How soon can you come get your mama?"

As Jon hung up the phone, thoughts flew through his head. "Memphis is 200 miles south of here. She hasn't been to Memphis in many years. How did Mom get down there? How do I get her home?"

Picking up the phone, he called his wife. "Honey, I know you're at a business meeting, but I need your help. Mom drove herself to Memphis and we need to go get her."

Jon's wife met him at home and Jon explained his plan. "It's eight o'clock now. If we leave now, we can be in Memphis before midnight. I can drive Mom's car and bring her home if you will drive my truck. We should be home around 4 A.M. I know you have to work tomorrow, and I'm sorry, but I need your help."

When Jon and his wife arrived in a poor midtown Memphis neighborhood, they found his mom in good health and spirits. She had knocked on the door of a kind, caring Memphis resident who allowed her to stay with her family all evening. The lady had fed her and treated her well. As

Jon, his wife and his mother were leaving, Jon told her, "I can't thank you enough for caring for my mother."

Jon asked his mother why she drove to Memphis. She replied, "I was going to the bank. Why would I go to Memphis?"

When Jon laid his head on the pillow that night, the questions whirled through his head: "Did Mom just make a wrong turn? How could she take a wrong turn, drive for four hours, and not realize something was wrong? Tomorrow I'll take her on her route to the bank and make sure she knows how to get there and return home."

Caregiving might begin dramatically with a big crisis, as it did with Jon's mother. Or it may begin quietly with a gut feeling that things just aren't right.

Mom can't remember how to change the channels on her new TV. "Understandable," we say. After all, new technology can be tricky to master. But months later, Mom still calls to say, "This TV isn't working right." When her son arrives to check on the TV, he finds Mom sitting and staring at a snowy screen, a channel with no reception. The son begins to worry. Is Mom really ok? Son lies awake at night, wondering what's happening to Mom's health.

Demographics

People live longer now. A baby boy born in 1900 had an average life expectancy of 46.3 years and a baby girl born in 1900 expected to live 48.3 years (all races in the U.S.). By comparison, a male born in 2005 can expect to live 75.2 years and a female 80.4 years (all races in the U.S.).[1] Life expectancy has been defined as the average number of years of life remaining at a given age. This increased life span has been attributed to improved public health.[2] In 1900, the leading causes of death were consumption (including tuberculosis) and pneumonia.[3] With the miracle drugs called antibiotics, many people now survive those past killers. In 2005 the leading causes of death were heart disease, cancer and stroke.[4]

Since 1900, increasing numbers of Americans live to age 65 and older. In 1900, 3.1 million (4.1 percent of the population) lived to be 65 or older. In 2009, 39.6 million (12.5 percent of the population) lived to be 65 or older.[5] With this increased life span and the increasing number of older Americans come the challenges faced by caregivers.

Caregiving Statistics

Sixty-five million people give care to chronically ill, elderly or disabled friends and family members every year. Caregiving involves many people: spouses, adult children — both sons and daughters, siblings, parents with sick children, even children who care for their parents and grandparents. Sixty-six percent of caregivers are women. Most commonly, an adult daughter, herself married and employed, provides care for her aging parent(s).[6] Caregivers may be raising their own children while helping aging parents, hence the term "sandwich generation."

Children also care for ill family members: "1.4 million children ages 8 to 18 provide care for an adult relative; 72 percent are caring for a parent or grandparent; and 64 percent live in the same household as their care recipient. Fortunately, most are not the sole caregiver."[7]

Parents dealing with a chronically ill child or a disabled child live with stress. The emotional roller coaster begins at the first indication that their baby has health concerns, and the parents are plunged from joyful anticipation to fear and concern.

Caregiver Economics

The care given to family and friends has a value of $375 billion a year, twice the amount spent on home-care and nursing home care ($158 billion). American caregivers spend an average of 20 hours per week caring for their family member. Thirteen percent of caregivers provide 40 hours or more of caregiving per week. While providing care caregivers find their caregiving responsibility interferes with work time and decreases their job income. In every state of the United States, families who have a disabled family member have a fifteen percent lower median income when compared to non-caregiving families. "During the 2009 economic downturn, 1 in 5 family caregivers had to move into the same home with their loved ones to cut expenses. 47% of working caregivers indicate an increase in caregiving expenses has caused them to use up all or most of their savings." Sixty percent of family caregivers are employed; however, caregiving has caused adjustments. Sixty-six percent of caregivers find they must adjust their work schedules and at times report to work late. Twenty percent of family caregivers have had to take a leave of absence from work. Caregivers and their families spend an average of $5531 annually on out-of-pocket expenses.[8]

Are You a Caregiver?

"Are you providing unpaid assistance to a spouse, relative or friend who is ill, disabled or needs help with basic activities of daily living? Do you help with rides to the doctor, shopping, meals, bill paying, bathing, grooming, dressing, walking or transferring to a wheelchair, housekeeping, managing medications, or arranging services to be provided by others? If you provide services like these, whether or not you live with the person you are helping, you are a caregiver."[9]

Short-term Caregiving vs. Long Term Caregiving

Raymond feels better and he's ready to get out of the hospital and resume life with his wife of 60 years. But wait. Their bossy daughters are still trying to tell him what to do. Don't they understand he's ready to take charge again? He's grateful for their help but they need to back off.

Short-term caregiving involves a specific short time frame and has a specific goal. An example of short-term caregiving would be a two-week vacation to care for Mom after her total knee replacement surgery. Short-term caregiving episodes often aren't too stressful for the caregiver and can be very rewarding.

Long-term caregiving stretches indefinitely into the future. The goals for long-term caregiving may not be obvious and they also may change. The goal may change from supporting Mom and Dad as they age to providing at-home, hospice end-of-life care after Mom dies and Dad, age 92, wants to finish out life at home. Long-term caregiving can grind on a person and wear him down into an exhausted, chronically stressed state.

Benefits of Caregiving

"Caregiving can be a gift in disguise — an experience that moves you toward a more meaningful connection with yourself and with others.... Service to others expands one's life and adds beauty."[10] Many people give care because they love and respect their ill family member. Caregivers find satisfaction in giving back to these significant persons — people who loved and nurtured them. Caregivers find meaning when they make a significant difference in their loved one's quality of life, and they provide a role model for their own children. A caregiver who has a positive attitude toward caregiving will receive greater benefits and satisfaction than a caregiver who feels trapped in the caregiving role or who feels bound by duty.

Dangers of Caregiving

How often have you seen it? Mrs. H has been sick for 10 years when all of a sudden her husband, Mr. H, dies. He never complained as he lovingly cared for Mrs. H every day. He appeared to be the healthy one of this couple. What happened to Mr. H?

Stress impacts the health of caregivers: "23% of family caregivers caring for loved ones for 5 years or more report their health is fair or poor." Eleven percent of family caregivers believe the caregiving situation has caused a deterioration of their own health.[11] Researchers have found caregiving stress can depress the caregiver's immune system and increase the risks of chronic illnesses. Caregiving stress can cause high blood pressure, anxiety, depression, and premature aging in caregivers: "Family caregivers experiencing extreme stress have been shown to age prematurely. This level of stress can take as much as 10 years off a family caregiver's life."[12]

Another danger of caregiving is isolation. The caregiver feels alone and wonders if they can accomplish the tasks ahead. Since we're social creatures, people need to feel loved and supported rather than isolated. Another danger occurs when a caregiver refuses help that's being offered — "No, I can do it." This reply slams the door on assistance with potentially dire consequences for the caregiver and the ill family member. This reply also cheats caring friends and support people of an opportunity to feel good after assisting this family.

Role reversals take place when the parent no longer can care of himself or his business. Mom can no longer write checks to pay bills and balance the checkbook. Dad can't hear well enough to navigate a voice-mail system at his doctor's office. They need help. The caregiver should give as much independence and dignity as possible to the elderly. The strong quiet father is forced by his frail aging body to accept help he doesn't want. The shrinking grey-haired mother is frightened that she forgets too many things. These elders must give up the family roles they've held for decades; their bodies have forced changes and indignities on them they never wanted.

Another role reversal occurs when the husband becomes ill. As his physical condition declines, he can no longer work, do chores or yard work. The wife becomes caregiver, sole wage-earner and handyman. During this transition, the wife may find herself grieving for the loss of her partner as she takes on more responsibilities. She's losing her lover and friend as her husband's health declines.

The Pasco-Pinellas County, Florida, Area Agency on Aging has identified four stages of caregiving:

Stage 1: When you become a Caregiver (starting at caregiving)
Stage 2: When you've been giving care for a while and need to find help
Stage 3: When you become a heavy-duty caregiver
Stage 4: When your caregiving duties are over and you have to let go.[13]

Caregiving Stages

People may not consider the early days of caregiving to be caregiving. When grandson mows Dad's yard every week, this help enables Dad to conserve his strength. When daughter spends her day off cleaning her parents' house and helping Mom get to the beauty shop, this conserves the strength and resources of Dad, who is primary caregiver. This timely support helps alleviate the weight of everyday life for aging parents and family members. Mom and Dad are still able to function in their world. Often the two aging spouses gradually decrease in strength and energy until the two halves can barely function as one whole person. Dad watches over Mom because he knows she will walk off and forget a pot cooking on the stove. When Dad's arthritis flares up, Mom snaps into a more alert state as she recognizes his physical need and responds.

Caregiving Stage 1

Acknowledge that caregiving has begun. As the ill person becomes more frail, more support and help are needed. Who will be the primary caregiver? Will the adult son who lives in town be primary caregiver? Will the nurse daughter receive this designation? How will caregiving responsibilities change the caregiver's life? Will siblings be able to come stay in town for respite (temporary relief for caregiver) vacations?

Respect the Care Receiver's Wishes

Well-meaning adult children sometimes take over more chores and responsibilities than the elderly parent is ready to relinquish. While talking with the parent, ask what he wants you to do.

1. Statistics and Stages of Caregiving

Dad wanted to die at home. It sounded good, but honoring his wishes became more and more difficult. After Mom died, he was lonely and sad. As they had been married for sixty years, family members expected him to grieve himself to death. He grieved deeply but he continued living for another 18 months after she died. As he passed his 91st birthday, Dad became more frail and unstable. He fell and hurt himself, bouncing off closet doors and the floor. His adult daughters wondered whether they should force him to move to a facility — "after all, he would have interaction with other people and help when he needed it." Although his body was frail, Dad's mind was alert and totally in control. He wanted to finish his life at home.

His three daughters wondered if they could manage this feat. His Arizona daughter came often and cared for him, giving support to her dad and respite to her sisters. The two daughters who lived close to him divided up the work. The daughter who lived a few blocks from their dad visited twice a day, before and after work, and became the first responder whenever Dad needed assistance and pushed his medical alert button. More than once she had to drop her work responsibilities to drive down the interstate eight miles and pick up Dad, who had fallen. This sister also served as Dad's power of attorney, handling all his bill paying and legal affairs. "Little sister" daughter came to visit every Saturday, bringing freshly cooked food, doing laundry and cleaning house. She walked away with her hands smelling like bleach and detergent. Grandchildren and extended family provided care and support. The support this family gave their dad and each other helped them survive this tough time.

How was it these three daughters could provide the help Dad needed? The answer: hospice services. A neighbor said that Dad would qualify for hospice services because of his heart failure. After a referral meeting with hospice staff, Dad and his family signed up. Hospice services provide care for terminally ill people. Hospice staff includes doctors, nurses, social workers, home health aides, chaplains, and volunteers. Hospice staff visited Dad several days every week, providing home health care and nursing assessment and supervision. Being a modest man, Dad had resisted his daughters' efforts to give him a shower, but he cooperated with the home health aide and began taking showers. Hospice staff helped obtain equipment Dad needed, such as a bedside commode and a hospital bed, which was set up in the living room of his small home. As the weeks passed, the three girls recognized that Dad's quality of life had improved greatly. They found the hospice staff always ready to answer questions and provide guidance.

As the months passed, Dad continued to weaken, and one Monday evening he had a heart attack. He experienced chest discomfort and shortness of breath. Coincidentally the hospice nurse stopped in and calmly assisted in making Dad comfortable. Over the next three weeks — Dad's last three weeks of life — the hospice staff gave guidance to the family: "Dad's heart condition is getting worse and he needs someone with him all the time. Does your family have a plan for this time?" The family had hired an experienced home health aide to check on Dad several times a day while the daughters were at work. At this time she began to stay with Dad all day and family members increased their time with Dad to provide the care he needed.

A Last Good-bye

A strong-willed man, Dad decided he was going to the family reunion scheduled for the next Sunday. His daughters thought he was crazy: "He can barely walk using his walker. How does he think he can attend the family reunion?" Despite their disbelief, they cooperated. The hospice nurse recognized Dad's plan to say good-bye to his only sister and his nieces and nephews, people he had loved for their entire lives. The hospice nurse made arrangements for a wheelchair and portable oxygen tank that Dad could use at the reunion.

His daughters watched Dad, through sheer willpower, pull himself up physically. The day before the reunion, Dad went into the kitchen and started opening cabinets. "Dad, what are you doing?" his daughter asked. "I'm making my cherry cheesecake for tomorrow," Dad said. "Why don't you sit at the bar and direct me while I make your dessert?" she offered. "No, I'll make it." When he finished making his cherry cheesecake, Dad was exhausted and returned to his bed.

Dad got up early the morning of the reunion. He shaved, got dressed and was returning to bed using his walker when his daughter awakened from her sleep on the couch. "You look nice, but what are you doing? It's 4 A.M." Dad said, "I'm ready for the reunion, but I'm going to lie down and rest."

During the reunion Dad enjoyed himself, visited with extended family and told them good-bye. A great nephew who shared a birthday and a special bond with Dad didn't want to hear it. He said, "I'll see you next year." Dad's daughter said, "No. He came today to say good-bye." When Dad left the reunion, he was exhausted. He had accomplished his task.

The next night Dad had another heart attack. The following day he lapsed into a coma and died with family at his side the following Friday.

Dad's family grieved but they also felt relief. They had honored Dad's wishes and he had died at home. They had gotten through this trying time by supporting and caring for each other and Dad.

Communicate

Communicate and communicate some more. Can a family meeting be arranged where everyone can talk about options and choices? If a sit-down meeting isn't possible, can e-mail or conference calling be utilized to accomplish this family meeting? If the elder care receiver is mentally competent, he should be included. This meeting may be emotional and difficult, especially if the elders or family members are in denial of the type and amount of help they need. Involving extended family members who want to help can provide tremendous support. The primary caregiver should not try to meet all the needs of the ill family member. It's not good for anyone. When possible, a group of family and friends should be supporting the ill elderly person. Family members can provide specific services such as lawn mowing and lawn care, weekly outings or routine doctor visits, or respite care for the primary caregiver's vacations. Friends and neighbors often offer to help. Instead of a vague "thanks but no thanks" response, caregivers should allow honest, reputable people (friends and neighbors) to assist by saying, "what would you like to do?"

What physical and mental conditions is the care receiver dealing with? A treatable thyroid problem, not Alzheimer's disease, may be causing Mom's recent memory loss. Mom should visit her doctor for an evaluation of recent changes. When a correct diagnosis is made, then family members can educate themselves on pertinent disease processes. The American Geriatric Society provides information on specific diseases at http://www.health inaging.org/agingintheknow/topics_trial.asp.

Making Memories

During the early stages of caregiving, many memories can be made and preserved. During this phase, audio and video tapes can be made and parents can share memories. Through all stages, pictures can be taken to preserve memories. One daughter spent time recording an audiotape of her father telling his life story. She now shares it with her children and grandchildren. The three-month-old great-great-grandson would not remember being held by the family patriarch but a picture will someday be used to show him his family heritage. One family made a family cookbook and included favorite pictures as well as Grandma's Cream of Tomato soup and Grandpa's Cherry Cheese Cake recipes.

Weekend days spent with Mom and Dad give companionship to all involved. Socializing over a hot casserole dish enables adult children to watch over the parents while enjoying time together. Family traditions can be passed on to the younger generations during these times.

Get Organized

During the early times, when Mom and Dad can make decisions regarding a will or trust, these legal documents should be brought up-to-date. A person may be appointed power of attorney (POA) to handle Mom and Dad's business when they're not able to do so. This POA can deposit Mom and Dad's checks and pay bills, etc., to keep legal and financial affairs up to date.

If Uncle John suffers a massive stroke and the doctors say there's no hope for recovery, what would he want done? Would he want to be kept alive indefinitely in a vegetative state? Would he want to be treated humanely but allowed to die naturally? A living will or durable power of attorney for Health Care (or both) ensures a person's wishes are followed. A living will states what John Doe wants done to him if he's unable to speak for himself. A "durable POA" document names the person John wants to make decisions about his health care if John cannot speak for himself. More information about POAs can be found in Chapter 8 of this book. Information about a durable POA for healthcare and a living will can be found in Chapter 6.

Create a notebook of information about the care receiver. The notebook could include a calendar with appointments, a list of medications, pertinent information about medical conditions or diet, and a list of pertinent phone numbers such as family members, friends, doctors, dentists and emergency contacts. This book will be useful when others are providing respite care for the caregivers.

What About Driving?

"I've been driving longer than you've lived." Ray became very defensive and angry when his adult daughter suggested it was time he stop driving. Americans love their cars and many an elderly person resists the suggestion to stop driving his. Families and friends can recognize the loss of independence and mobility, which may be felt emotionally by the elder person as a loss of control. However, physical deteriorations such as eyesight and coordination, perhaps caused by stroke, Parkinson's or dementia, may make aging drivers unsafe. Families can help in exploring alternative transportation sources to allow for independence.

Elder drivers and their families should consider the following situations as indications that driving may no longer be safe:

- If the driver cannot see over the dashboard or has difficulty reaching pedals or moving his foot from gas to brake pedal and vice versa
- If the driver no longer recognizes traffic signs and signals
- If the driver cannot turn to look over his shoulder
- If the driver has trouble hearing emergency sirens
- If the driver drives too fast or too slow compared to traffic
- If the driver forgets how to get to familiar places or is getting lost frequently
- If the driver cannot judge gaps between vehicles when merging or turning left
- If the driver becomes anxious, angry or confused when driving
- If the driver has been involved in an accident within the last couple of years or received more than one moving violation ticket within the last three years
- If other drivers often honk at him or frequently pass him on the right.[14]

Testing a person's driving skill can be accomplished through several ways. Many states' department of motor vehicle offices provide senior driving skill tests. Some rehabilitation centers offer safe driving assessments performed by occupational therapists. Vehicle adaptations might be needed for a senior driver capable of driving but who has a need for special equipment. The American Association of Retired Persons (AARP) "driving safely" program might be appropriate help for some senior drivers.

Home Safety

If living at home is a part of the plan, some modifications may be needed. Can the care receiver live on one floor? If not, can a family room or living room be turned into a bedroom? More information for making the home environment safe can be found in Chapter 8, "Practical Decisions."

Caregiving Stage 2: In for the Long Haul

Everyone recognizes that Dad's age (91) and frailty keep him from returning to independence and health. The best he can do is to shuffle to the bathroom and back. Dad falls often and sometimes he cannot get himself back up on his feet. Housekeeping and laundry are beyond his strength and energy. He needs meals provided. How can he continue living at home by himself? But that's his request — that he live at home until he dies.

Beth McLeon talks in her book *Caregiving* about the "independence trap." People equate maturity and strength of character with going it alone. She points out the mistake in this trap and recommends allowing others to assist in the caregiving.[15] A family meeting must be held. Resources should be utilized and help obtained. Caregivers are wise to utilize all resources to provide for the care receiver and themselves. The caregiving job is too large for any one individual. The single caregiver will wear out, burn out and become at risk for illness himself.

Give specific choices to people who offer to help. Family members may want to help but are unsure what is needed. An appropriate response might be, "We need a vacation this spring. Can you check your calendar and tell us when (March or April) you can come stay with Dad for a week?" Or "There's a tree hanging over Dad's garage and the limbs rest on the roof. Could you do some work on his yard and trees this spring? While you're here, we would get away for the weekend. What do you think?" Out-of-town family who want to provide financial support could give services such as lawn care, prepaid drug store cards, frozen meals, etc. Neighbors and friends may offer help. Have specific needs and give them choices of what they can do to help. Support from faith communities can be invaluable. Some faiths provide caregiver support groups. Senior programs are available at some churches. Caregivers interested in this support must communicate what they and their family need, whether physical, emotional and spiritual.

"Joining a support group is one of the best things you can do for yourself as a caregiver, truly a way to know that you are not alone."[16] Formal support groups exist for many diagnoses. For example, Alzheimer's support groups function in many cities and towns. These groups provide valuable information and a chance to share thoughts and feelings. Sometimes group members become extended family. They understand how a caregiver feels because they've been there and are still in that role. Social workers and chaplains at most hospitals can provide information and local phone numbers for support groups. Support groups can also be found through national organizations by calling toll-free phone numbers. Local Area Agency on Aging offices can give valuable sources of information and help. Nursing home facilities may have active support group programs.

Online support groups may be needed for some caregivers. Many reputable organizations provide online message boards or blogs to support caregivers. For example, the Alzheimer's Organization message board found at http://www.alz.org/living_with_alzheimers_message_boards_lwa.asp provides an online community and support group for both individuals and their caregivers. The National Family Caregivers Association message board can be accessed at http://www.nfcacares.org/connecting_caregivers/caregiver_message_boards.cfm.

Respite Care (Breaks from Caregiving)

Anyone involved with caregiving needs periodic breaks. These may be a few hours a week when the caregiver can pamper herself or take a walk in silence. It may be a week away to cruise the Caribbean, relaxing and rejuvenating both body and soul. Caregivers need times to recharge and relax. Those who don't take breaks away will cheat themselves as they risk burnout.

Caregivers Have Jobs

People providing care to family members also must deal with their jobs in the workplace. Over half of caregivers work full time. According to the U.S. Department of Labor, 30 percent of American workers give care to family members. Within ten years, that number is expected to rise to 54 percent.[17] Employed caregivers may find they're torn between their job and loyalty to their employer and their family member who needs them. While some companies offer nothing to the caregiver, other companies provide formal programs with resources and counseling. Some companies offer adult day care center services to employees and their families. Flexible scheduling, job sharing and telecommuting are policies which enable workers to fulfill their work duties while caring for loved ones.

The Family and Medical Leave Act of 1993 (FMLA) requires companies with 50 or more employees to offer up to twelve weeks of unpaid leave with job protection to employees for the following reasons: the birth and care of the newborn child of an employee; placement of an adopted or foster child to the employee; care of an immediate family member (spouse, child, or parent) with a serious health condition; or the employee who is unable to work because of his own serious health condition. The 2009 update to FMLA involves taking up to 26 weeks to care for a family member who is in the armed forces, National Guard or reserve and who is seriously ill.[18] Details of this update can be obtained at http://www.dol.gov/whd/fmla/finalrule/factsheet.pdf.

Stage 3: Heavy Duty Caregiving

Caregiving becomes more extensive as the care receiver's health declines. Caregiving duties may have been going on for a while already. Caregivers have two responsibilities at this time: to care for oneself and to protect the care receiver. Chapter 3, "Caregivers Need Care Too," and Chapter 4, "Stress Breakers," provide information for self care.

Provide What the Elderly Family Member Needs — Physical Needs

Caregivers and their support persons should periodically reevaluate what needs to be done. Mr. E's wandering took him outside and down the street on a cold winter night. His wife had fallen into an exhausted sleep and didn't know he was gone. Mr. E was found a few hours later by a neighbor coming home from work. Mr. E's distressed family recognized one person (his wife) couldn't keep up with him twenty-four hours a day and they moved him to an Alzheimer's secure facility.

How much care does the care receiver need? Later stages may mean picking up Dad when he falls and rehanging the closet door he knocked loose. It may mean assisting with his shower and learning to change dressings. Some portions of caregiving may feel awkward and emotional. An adult daughter may feel uncomfortable helping her dad take a shower. An adult son may not want to give his mother a suppository or an enema when she is constipated. One answer is garments which cover the person during a shower, which can be obtained at http://www.personalcarewear.com/. These "shower shield" garments preserve the person's modesty and dignity during showers and bathroom episodes and contribute to the emotional well-being of both caregiver and care receiver.

"One out of three adults 65 and older fall each year in the United States. Among those age 65 and older, falls are the leading cause of injury deaths. They are the most common cause of nonfatal injuries and hospital admissions for trauma. In 2007, over 18,000 older adults died from unintentional fall injuries." Men die from a fall more often than women, but women are more likely to have a nonfatal injury. As people age, their risk of being seriously injured increases.[19]

Dad didn't understand why the doctor recommended physical exercise after he fell several times. His doctor understood that exercising improves balance and increases strength, resulting in fewer falls. Fall prevention techniques include regular exercise. According to the Centers for Disease

Control and Prevention (CDC), other steps to prevent falling involve having a doctor or pharmacist review medications to avoid side effects and interactions which may cause dizziness or weakness. A yearly eye exam can detect failing vision which contributes to falls and injuries. As people age, they need brighter lights to see well.

Stage 4: Letting Go When Caregiving Duties Are Over

Dad looked at his oldest daughter and said, "I love you." Their relationship had often felt troubled and awkward; these final words he spoke to her brought healing to a life-long wound she carried.

The final stage of caregiving often involves the pain of letting go intermingled with heart-touching moments. Tasks for this stage include resolving relationships, making sure end-of-life decisions are complete, talking openly about death, considering hospice care, and continuing to care for self.[20] As Dad and his daughter did, many caregivers and care receivers are able to resolve emotional issues.

Forgiveness: Letting Go of Bitterness and Old Grudges

Caregivers deal with many emotions throughout. They may be angry at the care receiver or other family members. They may feel guilty because Mom's health required more care than they could accomplish at home. Caregivers may find forgiving to be an important, positive step during this stage. A caregiver may need to forgive the aging family member for past hurts and pain. A caregiver may need to forgive himself because he could no longer care for Mom and nursing home placement became necessary.

Forgiveness has been described as "a decision to let go of resentments and thoughts of revenge.... The act that hurt or offended you may always remain a part of your life. But forgiveness can lessen its grip on you and help you focus on other, positive parts of your life.... Forgiveness can even lead to feelings of understanding, empathy and compassion for the one who hurt you."[21] Researchers recognize that when a person holds onto anger, bitterness and grudges, that person may eventually have to deal with resulting long-term health problems. On the other side, forgiveness can provide benefits: decreased blood pressure, lower stress levels, less hostility, anxiety, chronic pain and depression, decreased alcohol and drug abuse and better anger management for the person who forgives.

Forgiveness happens when a person decides to forgive. The person who decides to forgive begins by recognizing how important forgiveness is and looking at the situation, how he reacted to the situation and how this reaction affected his life. Then the person chooses to forgive, moves away from victimhood and releases himself from "the control and power the offending person and situation have had in [his] life."[22]

Forgiveness requires effort but the results are better health and freedom from past pain. The person who forgives may or may not reconcile with the individual who hurt him. The hurtful individual may never change and may never apologize, but forgiveness takes the power away from the hurtful person and provides peace that helps you go on with life.[23] As one lets go of grudges, life will no longer be defined by hurt and victimhood.

Making end-of-life decisions and hospice care information can be found in Chapter 6. Readers can find information on grieving in Chapter 9. Through all stages of caregiving, caregivers must care for themselves while caring for their loved ones.

2

Children Involved in Caregiving

Children Who Need Care

Cindy, Jerry and Lindsey were anticipating the birth of a second child. After years of trying, Cindy and Jerry were thrilled at the idea of a second child. Their healthy three-year-old, Lindsey, was a joy, but they had room in their life for another child.

The pregnancy went along well. Mom felt fine and had no problems. At age 28, with no family history of any serious health issues, Cindy had every expectation that the child she carried would be healthy. An ultrasound test was normal and all seemed well. When it came time for their baby to be born, the delivery went fine and Mom and baby were ok.

Three hours after Ashley was born, joy turned to sorrow. The pediatrician called Jerry to a private room and said, "Don't tell your wife. Your daughter has Down syndrome." While Jerry's head was spinning, the doctor walked out, leaving him alone. When he could gather his composure, Jerry returned to his wife's room. She knew something was wrong. Jerry told Cindy, "The doctor said Ashley has Down syndrome."

The bottom fell out of their world. Cindy says "Of course, you could hear me screaming and crying a couple floors away. It was at least three more hours before we got to hold her or see her after we found that out. Hindsight, we wish we had her in our arms when we were told. Actually, with Down syndrome, it takes two weeks for the blood work to come back with results. At the time, it would have been nice if the news had been broken to us more gently. But that's not how it worked out."[1]

According to the Childstats.gov Website, "In 2005–2006, an estimated 14 percent of children ages 0–17 had a special health care need, as measured by parents' reports that their child had a health problem expected to last at least 12 months and which required prescription medication, more services than most children, special therapies, or which limited his or her ability to do things most children can do."[2] This group of special needs children and their families deal with health problems ranging from cerebral palsy to autism to childhood cancers, attention deficit hyperactivity disorders and a variety of other physical, mental and social problems.

How do these families begin to cope with the needs of their special needs child? Many, like Cindy and her family, begin by grieving. Later, Cindy spoke of it:

> It was the first time I've experienced depression and didn't realize that was what I was feeling. Whenever you give birth to a special needs child, you go through the same grieving process as if you would lose a child. I did not know that at the time. I went through the denial, I went through the anger; I went through all those steps. I remember I went to the library and got a book. I looked up the characteristics [of Down syndrome] and compared them to my daughter. Does she have that characteristic? Does she have the specks in her pupils? Does she have a crooked pinkie? I would take the book and checkmark every item in my effort to get some answers. But I definitely went through the grieving process as if losing a child. One day I heard Dr. James Dobson, *Focus on the Family*, talking on the radio. As I heard his words, it was like a bolt of lightning went through me. I was grieving the loss of my ideal child. This insight helped me deal with the feelings I had, the depression I felt, and the denial I had. The "I'll fix it; I'll find the right doctor to do the right thing" thought process. That was our biggest turning point. We realized we were ok; we were feeling things other people feel.[3]

Elizabeth Kubler-Ross became famous for her work with death and dying. She defined grief as having 5 stages: denial, anger, bargaining, depression and acceptance.[4] Denial says, "the doctor must be wrong. I don't believe it." Denial is a coping mechanism a person needs when the news he received is too painful. As he slowly begins to accept the news, this person's healing begins. Anger asks, "Why me? Why does my child have Down syndrome?" The second stage of grief, anger, is another coping mechanism. It covers the pain and gives socially acceptable strength to the pain. Bargaining says, "if only" or "what if." Bargaining tries to make deals: "If only the tests come back normal and my baby is healthy, I will do ____." During this stage, a person may want to stay in the past, in a more simple time. He may want to go back in time—before the special needs child was born and life became complicated. Depression says, "I will withdraw. I don't want to cope. Life is too painful and empty." This stage is appropriate and necessary at a time when a great loss has occurred. Acceptance says, "I see my daughter has special needs. How do we best help her?"

The five stages of grief do not always neatly progress in these five steps. There will be times when a person is plunged back into a prior stage, revisiting emotions and questions all over again. Not everyone goes through all stages, and not everyone spends the same amount of time in the different stages. Grieving is a personal experience.

Psychologist J. William Worden gives four tasks of mourning which a person can use to successfully get past the grief.[5]

Task 1 is to accept the reality of the loss. As Cindy said, she grieved the loss of her ideal child. "Coming to an acceptance of the reality of the loss takes time since it involves not only an intellectual acceptance but also an emotional one.... The bereaved person may be intellectually aware of the finality of the loss long before the emotions allow full acceptance of the information as true."[6]

Task 2 is to work through the pain of grief. Parents of special needs children know the pain and sorrow that Cindy and Jerry experienced: the joyful anticipation of a new baby that turns into sorrow and loss as they grapple with the new reality—the beloved child faces serious obstacles. Dr. Worden discusses a "literal physical pain that many people experience and the emotional and behavioral pain associated with loss.... It is impossible to lose someone you have been deeply attached to without experiencing some level of pain."[7] Healthy grieving includes recognizing this pain, allowing oneself to feel it and then dealing with it.

Task 3 is to adjust to an environment that has changed because of the loss. "The bereaved person searches for meaning in the loss and its attendant life changes in order to make sense of it and to regain some control of his or her life."[8] As Cindy and her family worked through their grief, she contacted a friend of a friend whose special needs child was amazingly successful, overcoming much of the cerebral palsy he was born with. When she contacted this family, they gave her insight into what had worked for them; they gave her phone numbers to get the help she needed.

Task 4 is to emotionally relocate the loss and move on with life. Dr. Worden warns this stage can be difficult. Some people "get stuck at this point in their grieving and later realize that their life in some way stopped at the point the loss occurred."[9] Cindy and her family worked through their grief and constructively turned their focus to what the youngest daughter needed. They had Ashley assessed as they moved into their new reality. They determined what Ashley needed and how to get those therapies and began working to maximize her chances of a successful development.

Families with a special needs child must begin to consider these questions: "What does my child need and where do I get those services?" One resource is the department of mental health each state has. The family can call and find out what's available there. A support group called MPACT (http://ptimpact.org/index.aspx) exists in several states and also can help.

Cindy gives insight into accessing help:

> The real life way to get services for your child is to find someone out there who has the same disability and connect with them. Someone who has already paved the way and made the phone calls can get you a lot further and quicker. I wish I could say there's a 1-800-wecare, but it's just not out there. It's sometimes difficult finding the services or the service is there but there's a waiting list. Families are the biggest resource. I think you also have to pick your battles and prioritize your child's needs. When we started therapy, what was important to us was physical therapy because babies learn so much the first year, growing, walking, and sitting so physical therapy was very important. Then speech therapy was very important because that's the next stage. Whenever my daughter got to the age where she needed preschool, we struggled to find a daycare or preschool that would accept a special needs child and would meet her needs, preparing her for kindergarten.[10]

Families with special needs children face increased financial stresses. When Cindy and Jerry had their daughter assessed, they discovered Ashley needed speech therapy, physical therapy and occupational therapy. She was put on a waiting list locally and they were told someone would call when an opening became available. Cindy called the St. Louis, Missouri, office (two hours away) and the staff at that office agreed Ashley needed all three therapies and said they could begin working with her the next week. Cindy said, "I quit my part time job, purchased a better car and drove Ashley to St. Louis for a year and a half—two days a week. My three-year-old, Lindsey, went to preschool for the first time so she wouldn't have to travel to St. Louis and watch therapies. That was a big life change for all of us: quitting my job, taking on extra finances, putting my older daughter in day care, traveling and doing therapy for six hours a day. After a year and a half, services became available locally, so we didn't have to commute back and forth."[11]

Families of special needs children face additional stress. Cindy attests to that fact:

In 1998 the state of Missouri divorce rate for families of special needs children was 98 percent. I'm not sure what the number is at present or statistics in other states. But parenting a special needs child puts extra stress on a marriage. Over the years several families with special needs children became our friends and support group. It's sad to know those families are no longer together. The stress of caring for a special needs child does wear on a relationship. The financial cost of a special needs child adds to the stress. Studies have shown that you will spend at least four more hours a day caring for that child than you would a typical child. You have a time issue, a finance issue and the heartache involved with a special needs child. If you're not careful, you'll take it out on your spouse. It takes a toll on marriages. If anything else comes along, it becomes "too much."[12]

How can families and friends help a family with a special needs child? Begin by loving and supporting them. Families and friends are their biggest resource. Be willing to listen to their joys and sorrows as they grapple with dealing with the new reality. Often a person doesn't know what to say in this situation. The experts recommend being supportive: "I want you to know I care." Offer real help, not vague offers: "What night next week can I bring supper for your family?" Sitting quietly with a person can give support. If he wants to talk, listen. If he doesn't talk, sit quietly. Many people aren't comfortable with silence, but caring silence can convey support.

Extended family members, including grandparents, may find themselves grieving for the child and for the parents: "The future is now unpredictable not only for the grandchild, but for the child's parents as well."[13] The family members may not recognize or acknowledge their emotions and find themselves coping on their own. Non-family members such as friends, neighbors and other people of the community can create stress: "Inability to cope with comments about the disorder or curious stares by others may foster the tendency to isolate and protect the child within the home."[14] One suggestion for parents is to minimize any differences by dressing the child as other children dress.

Recognize that some parents of special needs children may need time to grieve. Cindy and Jerry felt this grief because all their hopes and dreams for their ideal second child flew out the window when they were told she had Down syndrome. They felt the same grief and sorrow as if she had died, but she was very much alive and needed their love and care. Cindy talked about this sorrow: "In this situation you don't have a burial that you would have with a child that you really did lose. You don't have the sorrow or the sympathy or even the closure that you would have. It was something very personal and very lonely. Nobody else would recognize that—or even know how to help or console. I don't think most of our family recognized that we were grieving as if we had lost a child."[15] Family and friends who want to give practical help might provide meals and help with child care when appropriate. Many couples would welcome a respite, a relaxing time away from the care of their child. Caring family and friends can find many ways to love and support the couple and their children.

There is upbeat news from Cindy and Jerry's household. The couple worked through the challenges to keep their marriage alive and their family intact. They've had a third child, now a healthy five-year-old, a daughter named Abigail. At age 16, Ashley is a freshman in high school who does well in her classes, especially in math. Recently Ashley brought a St. Louis newspaper to her mom. "Look Mom," she said, "the Jonas Brothers are going to be in St. Louis for a concert." Cindy continues: "Ashley read the date, time and how much the tickets cost with a plea of 'can we go, Mom.'"[16]

Cindy and Jerry expect that Ashley will be a self-sufficient person as an adult. They attribute much of her high function and success to the early therapies and all the hard work their family has invested into Ashley's physical, mental, spiritual, and social education.

Children Who Give Care

Children are not small adults. They have growing and learning to do before adult responsibilities are thrust upon them. However, children may find themselves in a caregiving role. Cindy Brotherton tells how their five-year-old daughter, Abigail, often offers to help her sixteen-year-old "big sister" Ashley. "She's always saying, 'I'll help you, sister. I'll get that for you.' We have to intervene a lot because we want Abigail to enjoy her childhood and not become burdened by caregiving duties."[17]

Thirty-one percent of the children who act as caregivers are ages eight to eleven, 38 percent are ages 12 to 15 and the remaining 31 percent are ages 16 to 18. These young caregivers provide care to a parent, grandparent or sibling and two-thirds of them live in the same household as the care receiver. Most commonly, the care recipients have Alzheimer's or other dementia, diseases of the heart, lung or kidneys, arthritis or diabetes.

These young caregivers spend time keeping their loved one company (96 percent) and helping with chores (85 percent). Sixty-five percent grocery shop and 63 percent prepare meals for their loved one. Fifty-eight percent of these young caregivers help their loved one with one or more activity of daily living (ADL) such as bathing, dressing, toileting, and feeding.[18]

How do these young caregivers fare? "Overall, caregivers' feelings of self-esteem, sadness, loneliness, and fun are similar to those of non-caregivers. However, boy caregivers are more likely to feel sad than are boys who are not caregivers (52% vs. 38%)."[19] Both caregivers and non-caregivers report school problems in similar numbers. Experts believe young caregivers are more likely to have problems when they live in the same household with the ill elderly family member, when they perform personal care tasks for the loved one and when they're a minority household.

When a significant adult in a child's life, especially a parent, becomes critically ill, that child may feel responsible and worry that the parent will die. Other family members may be overwhelmed and forget that children may be worried. An unexpected hospitalization or illness may cause stress to the children of the family. The kids may find themselves staying with relatives and dealing with unfamiliar routines. They may miss time with both parents, the ill parent, who is undergoing medical treatments, and the caregiving parent, who is suddenly overwhelmed with the medical crisis. Children may begin showing signs of stress, such as a shortened attention span or plummeting grades. The stressed child may act sullen, withdrawn or sad and may ask questions about whether other family members, and even he, will stay healthy or get sick and die.

The first step in helping children cope with family illness is to recognize that they need to know what's going on. "They need to know that they are not responsible for the adult's or sibling's condition.... Providing simple and understandable information about the condition, and answering their questions, goes a long way to resolving guilt feelings, as well as easing fear based on the unknown."[20] False reassurances like "there's nothing to worry about" when there truly are serious problems can decrease the child's trust in the adults who are saying that. It's better to explain in simple but honest terms like "Mommy is sick. She's going to the doctor next week. We will give you more information when we know something."

Even children who appear to be coping well with family sickness need attention. An offer to take a child to visit the sick parent/grandparent in the hospital will be an opportunity to reassure the child. However, if the sick parent/grandparent is critically ill, the child should be prepared by the adults for what he will see. In this situation, the adults may choose not to take the child to visit.

Another helpful suggestion involves keeping to normal routines.

Children find comfort and security in familiar routines such as homework, playtime and chores. These children need love and attention the same (if not more) as if everyone in the household were healthy.[21]

Children grieve just as adults do: "Grief is not limited to death and divorce; life changes of every kind can elicit a grief response which is just as powerful in children as in adults, and is generally less understood."[22] The Harvard Child Bereavement Study followed 125 children (ages 6 to 17) for two years after the death of a parent. In 74 percent of the families the father had died. Twenty-six percent of the families had lost a mother to death. The researchers found that the death of the mother affected the children more than the death of the father for two reasons: their daily routines changed and the emotional caretaker (the mother) was absent.[23]

The researchers found that "children doing well tended to come from more cohesive families, where communication about the dead parent was easy, and where fewer daily life changes and disruptions took place.... Three things children need after the death of a parent are support, nurturance (affection and caring), and continuity (uninterrupted routines and behaviors)."[24] Adults can help the children cope by keeping their normal routines, being consistent and loving and allowing them to talk about their feelings. The parent should reassure the children that they will be cared for and let them know they're not responsible for their parent's death as well as what caused the death. The researchers found that children benefited from being involved in decisions about the funeral of their parent (or at least being asked if they want to help make decisions): "Bereaved children need ways to remember the dead person."[25] The author recommends that a memory book/picture album be made as a family project to give the child a tangible memory.

Widowed parents may wonder if and when they should start to date again. The researchers found that "parental dating in the first year of bereavement was associated with withdrawn behavior, acting out behavior, and somatic (physical) symptoms, especially if the parent was a father. The effects of engagement or remarriage after a suitable bereavement period had a positive influence on the children, leading to less anxiety, depression and worry about the safety of the surviving parent."[26]

Adults who recognize that children involved with caregiving deal with stress and grief can help the kids find ways to cope constructively. Adults must recognize that each child is a unique individual and should be treated as such. Social workers and teachers can often give insight into how best to support these children during their caregiving time. If a sibling becomes ill or is born with problems, other children in the home should be supported. Suggested behaviors involve promoting healthy sibling relationships, helping siblings cope and involve siblings.[27]

Promoting healthy sibling relationships begins with valuing each child as an individual. Parents should cheer for their children's successes and show the healthy child how to interact with the sibling. They should give the healthy child freedom to have activities separate from the special needs child. Letting children settle their differences, providing no one is in danger of being hurt, helps support both healthy and special needs children.

Helping siblings cope begins with listening. Parents should praise the healthy sibling for positive behaviors such as being patient with the special needs child or being helpful. Parents can talk with teachers and ask for their support. If a parent is alert, he can often recognize times of stress for the healthy child and support that child. When needed, social workers or counselors can help support the healthy sibling. Parents can involve a sibling in the life of the special needs child without burdening him with the work. If support groups for siblings are available, this resource might be tremendously supportive. Parents can include siblings by teaching them about the special needs child's illness, treatment plans and future goals.[28]

Developmental Stages of Childhood

Physical development of childhood begins at conception and continues through the teenage years until adulthood. During this almost twenty-year span, a fertilized egg becomes a baby who grows physically, mentally, emotionally and spiritually through the stages of life and becomes a young adult. The developmental age periods are often divided into prenatal, infancy, early childhood, middle childhood, and later childhood. When parents recognize the normal developmental stages of childhood, they can foster their child's growth in healthy, normal ways.

The Prenatal period begins at conception and continues through birth. This period of cell differentiation and rapid growth is a very important time in the life of a child. The health and nutritional status of the mother impacts the child's health during this period. All pregnant women should receive prenatal care from a physician or a nurse practitioner/midwife trained in the care of pregnant women.

Infancy begins at birth and continues through the first twelve months of a child's life. Rapid changes occur as a baby grows and matures. Birth weight usually triples during those twelve months. The baby grows longer, averaging a 50 percent length increase. The child develops physically as he first becomes strong enough to control his head movements. As the months progress, most babies roll over, crawl and finally walk.

The psychosocial development (Erikson) during this time involves trust: "Consistent, loving care by a mothering person is essential to development of trust."[29] If the child doesn't receive loving care, mistrust begins that may affect the child throughout his life.

Early childhood encompasses the years from one to six. The years one to three are called toddler years and the years three to six are preschool years. During these years children go from their first steps to running as motor development continues, they develop language skills and social relationships.

The psychosocial work of the toddler years involves autonomy (functioning independently). Toddlers strive to attain independence as they say "no" and "me do it." Toddlers want to do things for themselves and they learn much from imitating the behaviors they see. Parents of toddlers will better cope with what may be seen as frustrating behavior when they recognize this is normal work for their child. The positive outcome of this stage involves self-control and will power. The negative side can be doubt and shame if children are belittled or if they're forced to be dependent about things they can control.[30]

The psychosocial work of preschool children (ages 3 to 6 years) involves initiative — the ability to start on a new idea. During this time children develop a conscience, a sense of right and wrong with the desire to do right. Children explore their world using all their senses and powers. A positive outcome gives them direction and purpose. A negative outcome results in feelings of guilt. "Children sometimes undertake goals or activities that are in conflict with those of parents or others, and being made to feel that their activities or imaginings are bad produces a sense of guilt. Children must learn to retain a sense of initiative without impinging on the rights and privileges of others."[31]

Middle childhood or school age years includes 6 to 11 years of age, when physical development continues. During these years, a child's world enlarges greatly as he goes to school and enters the world of peer pressure.

The psychosocial work of middle childhood involves industry. Children want to be busy; they want to accomplish their tasks and be successful. They are "ready to be workers and producers."[32] During this time, children learn to compete as well as cooperate. They learn the rules. The positive outcome of this stage is competence. The negative outcome, inferiority, results when a child begins to feel like a failure who is unable to meet the standards set for them by others.

Later childhood involves ages 12 to 19. This period is often divided into prepubertal (years 12 and 13) and adolescence (years 13 through 19). Tremendous physical changes occur during these years as bodies change and grow into more adult sizes and shapes.

Psychosocial work of this age group involves identity: "Who am I? What do I want to be in my life?" Peer pressure becomes increasingly important. Teenagers become preoccupied with how others see them vs. their self-concept. As teens struggle to become independent of parents and home, they find a group of peers to join. During these years, teens struggle with boyfriend and girlfriend issues and enter the dating world. Their future career and education for their life's work become important. Positive outcomes involve devotion to their beliefs and values and the people they love. Role confusion, the negative outcome, happens if teens cannot resolve the identity issue.[33]

Children are important members of their families. As such, children may be involved in caregiving, either as a recipient or as a giver. Children with special needs require extra care from their families. A significant number of children give care to family members. Caregiving by children can be helpful to the family and beneficial to the children themselves if they aren't overburdened with chores. The healthy adult family members should remember that children have developmental work they must do. When children accomplish their developmental tasks, they will grow up healthy, mentally, psychologically and socially.

3

Caregivers Need Care Too

"These caregivers are on a path seemingly without end, subjected to the stresses and the guilts of watching another's pain without being able to erase it, of witnessing a loved one's dying without being able to prevent it. They quietly sacrifice personal agendas to look after those in need, often sandwiched between child care and jobs and usually without advance planning. They live a world apart from everyday reality and wonder if they will ever be normal again. They have one goal: to maintain the dignity and the well-being of their loved one until the end."[1]

Dad deserves a better epitaph than this: "Dad got the best of care, while we became tired, sick and depressed." Too many caregivers trudge ahead day after day, not caring for self at a most challenging time of life. They need to care for themselves while maintaining the "dignity and well-being of their loved one." "First, care for yourself.... When your needs are taken care of, the person you care for will benefit, too." This advice comes from the Family Caregiver Alliance.[2] The American Heart Association says, "If you don't pace yourself, you're going to be depleted before the job is done. Think of caregiving as a marathon, not a sprint. Marathoners get through a race by pacing themselves and getting sustenance and water along the way."[3]

Stress

Stress has been called the number one threat to a caregiver's health. The chronic ongoing stress of caregiving wears on people and can lead to symptoms of high blood pressure, arthritis flare-ups, acid reflux, sleeplessness, headaches, chronic back pain, and muscle aches. According to a National Academy of Sciences report, a caregiver of a person diagnosed with dementia finds his own immune system depressed for up to three years after the caregiving ends. This depressed immune system contributes to chronic illness for the caregiver. A caregiver can even find his own life shortened, as the extreme stresses of caregiving can "take as many as 10 years off a family caregiver's life."[4]

Stress is defined as "mental or physical tension." All people feel stress, but whether they perceive a situation as stressful and how much they react to it varies. For example, one person may shudder in fear when he is asked to make a speech while another individual thrives as a public speaker.

The human response to stress can be traced back to prehistoric man. When he met a tiger or bear, he recognized the danger and his body responded with the "fight or flight" response. Two types of chemicals, catecholamines (dopamine, norepinephrine and epinephrine) and steroid hormones, were released. These chemicals prepared his body to run away or fight. The body's blood supply was diverted to vital organs such as the heart, lungs and skeletal muscles and resulted in increased heart rate, breathing, and muscle tension, priming his body for action. In modern-day societies, few people encounter tigers and bears. However, the same stress response occurs when daughter's phone rings with a message from the medic alert staff that her Dad has fallen and can't get up. His daughter must leave work, rushing through traffic to get him up off the floor. When stress occurs frequently and for a long period of time, it wears people down physically, mentally and emotionally.

Research published in the February 2009 issue of the proceedings of the National Academy of Sciences points to an explanation for this. Scientists found that brief increases of stress hormones enhanced energy production at the cellular level (in the mitochondria), while high doses or long-term levels of these hormones depressed the function of the mitochondria. Researchers believe stress hormones "boost mitochondrial functions to provide cells with more energy for coping with and adapting to acute challenges.... However, chronic stress may lead to chronically elevated levels of glucocorticoids, which in turn may reduce cell functioning."[5]

Research has shown that people dealing with chronic stress heal their wounds more slowly and face increased risk of catching colds and flu when they are exposed. Experts believe that the brains of chronically stressed people start to shrink and connections between brain cells are damaged, which may explain the memory problems, decreased focus, and problem-solving skills some of those individuals experience.[6]

Caregivers Need Care Too

The National Family Caregiver Association offers the following tips to cope with stress: "speak up ... learn to say 'yes' to offers of help ... create a social network ... watch your own health ... give yourself a break ... review your loved one's health coverage ... seek expert advice."[7]

Caregivers Need Physical Care

Caregivers often overlook their own health needs. When their schedule fills up with Mom's appointments and picking up prescriptions, they delay their own yearly medical and dental checkups. Caregivers must put their own physical well-being at the top of their priority list. What physical needs should caregivers attend to? Caregivers should talk to their doctors to set up an individualized plan for themselves.

According to the Mayo Clinic, the top two health threats for both men and women are heart disease and cancer.[8] For many years, everyone thought that men lived with a higher risk of heart disease than women. Not true. One in three men and women in America deals with cardiovascular disease, including myocardial infarction (MI or heart attack), strokes, congestive heart failure, and congenital heart problems. Coronary heart disease is the number one killer of Americans.

What can a person do to decrease his risk of heart disease? The experts at the Mayo Clinic and the American Heart Association offer advice: improve diet, keep weight within normal range, add exercise to the daily routine, avoid smoking and tobacco products, drink alcohol in moderation and work with a doctor to keep blood pressure, diabetes and blood cholesterol levels within normal limits.

Overstressed caregivers can easily find themselves turning to comfort foods and falling into bad habits such as smoking or drinking and leaving off exercise. When the caregiver recognizes this behavior, he can modify it. If he takes charge and changes one thing, he will feel a sense of accomplishment and control. By taking a walk on a warm spring day, the caregiver can enjoy the splashes of color in blooming daffodils and cherry trees while lowering his stress levels.

The number two health risk to Americans is cancer. Prostate cancer, lung cancer and colorectal cancer rank as the top three types of cancer in American men. For American women the top three types of cancer causing death are breast cancer, lung cancer and colorectal cancer. The American Cancer Society points out that "one third of all cancer deaths are related to poor diet, physical inactivity and carrying excess weight." They advocate control of one's weight, a healthy diet and physical activity as cancer prevention strategies. These experts believe a person's "excess weight causes the body to produce and circulate more of the hormones estrogen and insulin, which can stimulate cancer growth."[9]

Caregivers should protect their own health. The National Family Caregivers Association says it well: "The best present you can give your loved one: your own good health." They recommend daily care that includes a vitamin supplement and brushing and flossing teeth. Weekly care includes exercising and talking with a support buddy or group. Each month the caregiver should get away for fun, and add spirituality if he chooses to do so. On a yearly basis, caregivers should get a flu vaccine, see their doctors for an annual physical and take a respite vacation away from the cares and responsibilities of caregiving.[10] During the annual physical, a person and his doctor should discuss and schedule preventive tests such as mammograms, pelvic exams, colon cancer screening, hearing and vision tests and bone density studies as the doctor recommends.

The Administration of Aging recommends an additional two vaccinations: pneumococcal pneumonia and tetanus (lockjaw): "Influenza and pneumonia are the fifth leading cause of death in older adults. More than 90% of those who die from flu and pneumonia are people 65 years of age and older. Tetanus, although rare, tends more often to be fatal for older adults."[11] The pneumococcal vaccine is a one time immunization, unless a booster shot is recommended for high-risk people. The tetanus-diphtheria (Td) vaccine protects against tetanus and diphtheria and a booster shot for tetanus-diphtheria is recommended every 10 years.

What can caregivers do to better deal with this stress? A sense of being in control is one factor in whether or not humans feel stressed.[12] Caregivers find many things beyond their control. Aging parents may need increasing amounts of help but continue to be in control, bumping heads with their adult children caregivers. These caregivers can decide to pick the important battles while trying to ignore the minor issues and honor their parent's wishes. If the aging parent is mentally competent, his decisions are legal and should be honored. The caregiver can decrease his stress by choosing not to worry about things beyond his control.

"Your attitude can be the biggest barrier to taking care of yourself and doing the best job for your loved one." According to the American Heart Association Web page Reality Check, one of the few things a caregiver can control is his own response to the situation. "Your mind will believe what you tell it. Tell it that you're a caregiver, that you need to stay healthy, that you have rights and that you will do the best you can but you'll have to find help for certain things."[13]

Caregivers Need Emotional Care

"Family caregiving is an emotional roller coaster that can leave a person exhausted, bewildered, and dislodged, wondering how she or he can feel so helpless in a period so supposedly grown-up."[14] Caregivers deal with emotions. They may feel love for the sweet little mother and sadness because she's becoming frail. They may feel frustrated that all their efforts "couldn't put Humpty together again." They may feel anger and resentment that no one comes to visit Mom and guilt when they become exhausted and cannot give anymore. Caregiving becomes a very emotional time. It's no wonder caregivers become sad and depressed: "40 to 70 percent of family caregivers have clinically significant symptoms of depression with approximately a quarter to half of these caregivers meeting the diagnostic criteria for major depression."[15]

Worry is an emotion in which a person feels anxious or concerned about a real or imagined issue. Anxiety adds a physical response to the emotion of worry. These symptoms include sweating, increased heart rate or palpitations, and elevated blood pressure. Both worry and anxiety are normal and may even be productive if they spur a person to prepare and cope better. For example, a student worried about keeping a good grade will probably study and score better on the test than if he didn't study. But when they are excessive, both worry and anxiety become harmful to people.

Depression is a condition marked by feelings of hopelessness, self-doubt, and lethargy. Caregivers suffer from depression symptoms at more than twice the rate of the general population.[16] "Depression is a serious medical condition that affects the body, mood and thoughts. It affects the way one eats and sleeps, one's self concept, and the way one thinks about things. A depressive disorder is not the same as a passing blue mood. It is not a sign of personal weakness or a condition that can be willed or wished away.... Appropriate treatment, however, often involving medication and/or short term psychotherapy, can help most people who suffer from depression."[17]

When a person is stressed, he may display both emotional and behavioral symptoms which can include nervousness, anxiety, changes in eating habits (either overeating or not eating enough), loss of energy, and mood chances.

Caregivers Need Social Support

Where should caregivers seek social support? Researcher Dr. Shelley E. Taylor analyzed 216 scientific studies and noted some differences in how men and women respond to stress. Historically, men as the larger and stronger of the species, tended to react more aggressively to stress. Women often could neither run nor fight because their children needed care. Through the ages, women found that tending and soothing their children resulted in decreased stress levels. The female hormones oxytocin, and possibly estrogen, may contribute to the female's more social needs and responses during stressful times.

Dr. Taylor's research points to social support as being important during stressful times. Both men and women, but especially women, gain tremendous social support from women. In fact, Dr. Taylor believes women seek support from their female friends in time of stress: "Social support has stronger effects on women's health outcomes than on men's." Her conclusion, "fight-or-flight more descriptive of men; tend and befriend more descriptive of women's stress responses. Men receive [much of their] social support from women; women receive [much of their] social support from other women. As such, women's ties with other women promote health and longevity."[18]

Caregivers Need Spiritual Care

"A Columbia University study found that people who make religion a significant part of their lives are 81% less likely to battle anxiety and depression and are more likely to have confidence that they can recover from an illness."[19] A 2004 survey of Americans showed that "45% had used prayer for health reasons, 43% had prayed for their own health, almost 25% had had others pray for them, and almost 10% had participated in a prayer group for their health."[20]

Sue Wessel shares these thoughts after her caregiving experiences: "Not only do we have Mom, but we both work stressful jobs. We have our own immediate family that I worry about. I have a 30 and 34 year old that I worry about. I lay in bed worrying about them (our children) and I think about what I forgot to do at work. I've got Mom lying in the next room. I worry that's she's going to get up some night and fall. Sometimes I just have to say, 'Lord, it's yours.' Give it to him. Do my best and give it to him."[21]

Researchers wonder whether prayer accomplishes better coping with stress and improved health or whether there's an actual physical change from prayer. Researchers at Memorial Sloan-Kettering Cancer Center published a study in 2003 which concluded that spiritual well-being protects a person from the sadness and despair associated with end-of-life events. These researchers are working to measure spirituality and levels of interleukin-6 (IL-6) among terminally ill cancer patients: "There is a small, but growing, body of literature linking immune function to mood, and IL-6 is the immune marker most highly correlated with mood states."[22]

WebMD.com's Caregiver tip #1 is this: Caregivers must take care of self first.[23] If caregivers do not put self first, they will exhaust themselves, running out of resources needed to care for their loved one. They can suffer from burnout. Signs and symptoms of caregiver burnout include crying a lot, feeling helpless or hopeless, overreacting to minor situations, feeling exhausted or overwhelmed, losing interest in work and being less productive, changes in normal eating or sleeping habits, being unable to relax, being short-tempered, withdrawing from people, increasingly thinking of death, and taking larger doses or more frequent medications for insomnia, anxiety or depression.[24]

The caregiver who has multiple stresses would be at increased risk for burnout. For example, a caregiver could easily feel overwhelmed if her 91-year-old father has terminal cancer, and her 86-year-old mother-in-law who wandered away from home is subsequently diagnosed with Alzheimer's disease, all while this caregiver is dealing with a stressful project at work.

Other causes of caregiver burnout include role confusion and unrealistic expectations. When a sudden illness causes one spouse to become caregiver to the other, role confusion can occur. No longer just his wife, she now must provide care for her husband while taking care of chores he used to do, such as paying the bills and yard work.

Caregivers may also deal with unrealistic expectations. The daughter working to obtain the best medical care for her parents may find it painful watching their health slip away. All her efforts cannot regain her parents' health or turn back the clock on their advancing ages. These unrealistic expectations can contribute to frustration and caregiver burnout.

Strategies for "Avoiding Burnout During Caregiving" can be found at http://www.caps4caregivers.org/Assets/CAPSsummer2007B.pdf. Valuable suggestions include keeping in touch with friends and accepting their love and support, learning relaxation techniques, taking time to care for your own health, keeping a life outside your caregiving role, building a caregiving team utilizing the help of professionals, relying on a sense of humor, and finding a support group either online or in person where you can feel supported and share your feelings.[25]

Caregivers Can Take Care of Self

According to WebMD authorities, caregivers should set aside time every day for self. Each person should spend this free time doing something pleasurable — reading a fun book, taking a walk during a sunshiny day, or meditating quietly. See chapter 4 for suggestions of pleasurable, de-stressing techniques and activities

Readers may notice the consistent recommendations from caregiver groups, the American Heart Association, and the American Cancer Society: take care of self, eat healthy food, exercise, add pleasure back to life, accept help with caregiving responsibilities and utilize support from friends, families, and official support groups.

Get Enough Sleep

"Insomnia is the most common sleep complaint among Americans.... There's a wealth of research indicating that people with insomnia have poorer overall health, more work absenteeism and a higher incidence of depression."[26] According to 2009 survey conducted by the National Sleep Foundation, "one-third of Americans are losing sleep over the state of the U.S. economy and other personal financial concerns." Caregivers may find themselves worrying about economic issues even in good financial times. Over the past eight years, the number of Americans sleeping less than six hours a night changed from 13 to 20 percent. Fewer people (from 38 percent to 28 percent) get eight hours or more sleep per night.[27]

People dealing with insomnia should begin with a talk with their doctor. Some medications such as those for colds and allergy, high blood pressure and heart disease, thyroid disease, asthma, pain, birth control and depression (especially SSRI antidepressants) can cause insomnia. The National Sleep Foundation, at www.sleepfoundation.org, provides suggestions people can utilize in their search for a good night's sleep.

Eat Healthily

Nutrients from food are what the human body uses to rebuild and repair. A balanced diet of carbohydrates, proteins and fats, vitamins and minerals provide fuel and building blocks the body needs to stay healthy. The experts at the American Association of Retired Persons (AARP) suggest "now more than ever, try to eat regular, light meals that feature whole grains, fruits and vegetables, and low-fat meats and cheeses. Make an effort to limit your intake of saturated fats and sugars. Be particularly careful about self-medicating with too much alcohol and coffee."[28] Current recommendations by the American Dietetic Association for a healthy diet can be accessed at www.eatright.org. The U.S. Department of Agriculture provides information about a healthy diet at www.choosemyplate.com.

When people face a big stress, the "fight or flight" hormones are released and the body primes itself to fight or run away. During that time, appetite for food will decrease. In the next phase, the slower moving cortisol (stress hormone) kicks in and the appetite for food increases. Scientists believe a feedback system exists to turn off the stress hormones but that chronic stress alters this system and it doesn't turn off. Based on studies of rats, chronic and constant stresses continue a cycle that never shuts down. The rats continue to eat high sugar, high fat foods and develop abdominal obesity and related health problems. Scientists believe humans react in a similar manner.[29]

Exercise

Caregivers may feel too tired or stressed to consider exercise. A caregiver could say that, after working all day, running by Mom's house to check on her, and hurrying home to feed the kids before the evening's soccer game, she doesn't have the time or energy to exercise.

The 2000 Family Caregivers Survey confirms the problem. It shows that the number of family caregivers who exercised regularly dropped when they became caregivers. Before caregiving, 61 percent exercised regularly, while 30 percent exercised regularly afterwards.[30] Yet exercise has been proven beneficial. The American Heart Association says physical exercise "tackles anxiety, depression and anger. It enhances your immune system and decreases the risk of developing disease such as cancer and heart disease. It helps maintain a healthy weight.... For each hour of regular exercise you get, you'll gain about two hours of life expectancy, even if you don't start until middle age."[31] Other benefits include helping prevent bone loss, reducing the risk of heart disease, and improving muscle strength, energy levels and sleep. "Three 10-minute periods of activity are almost as beneficial to your overall fitness as one 30-minute session."[32]

A study held at Stanford University recruited 100 postmenopausal caregiving women to measure how exercise would affect their stress levels. These women were caring for a spouse or relative with Alzheimer's disease or another type of dementia and averaged 72 hours per week in caregiving activities. Half of these women exercised for 30 minutes four times a week and kept an exercise log. The non-exercise women in the study were giving information on how to follow a low-fat, heart healthy diet. "The biggest improvements appeared to be in how the participants dealt with stress.... Those in the exercise group reported a marked improvement in the quality of their sleep, as well as lower blood pressure reactivity levels in response to stressful situations."[33] Caregivers should consider exercise a gift of health to themselves, a valuable investment in their mental and physical health.

Add Pleasure Back to Life

Forget the guilt. Caregivers can become overwhelmed with guilt. "Wallowing in disappointment over something you did is not productive.... Carrying the burden of disappointment in yourself or in others is something we choose to do and something we would not do if we had our health in mind."[34] Caregivers can choose to forgive self and others and leave that load behind. "Feelings of guilt, according to a study by doctors at the University of Hull in England, interfere with the body's production of the antibody immunoglobulin A, which protects against infection."[35]

Laugh

"Laughter helps us deal with pain and difficulties and is valuable in a medical context because it reduces our anxiety and our body's state of alarm. Take time out when you are sick or worried about your health to watch your favorite comedy or read your favorite amusing book."[36] More information can be found in chapter 4, in the "Humor" section.

Need a Hug?

Many people go through their day needing a caring, friendly touch. "Everybody needs a daily dose of attention and a daily dose of touch for their emotional well-being. It is as important as diet and exercise." Researchers have found that a brief hug from a loved one decreases the effects of stress on heart rate and blood pressure by half.[37]

Prescription Medications

Caregivers may find they need antidepressant medications. When the cares and sorrows of caregiving add too much stress and sadness to life, these medications may help immensely. A conversation with a physician can reveal appropriate medications for each individual case.

Accept Help with Caregiving Responsibilities from Family, Friends, and Support Groups

"Caregivers who relied upon the support of friends, family, or support groups to help them deal with the emotional burden of caregiving were 59% less likely to report feeling overwhelmed by their responsibilities than were those who faced caregiving alone."[38] Local support groups can be found through social workers at hospitals and through the local Area Agencies on Aging http://www.eldercare.gov/. Reputable online support groups can be found through organizations. For example, the Alzheimer's Association can be accessed at www.alz.org.

Primary Caregiver Role

At first, perhaps, the parents only need someone to care for the outside chores, such as mowing the grass. As they become more fragile, increasing amounts of help are needed. Usually one person becomes the primary caregiver, whether by geographic proximity, age or emotional ties. As this person becomes more involved in caregiving, that individual may resent this unequal weight of responsibility. Out-of-town family members can step up and shoulder some of the load, avoiding an uneven burden on the primary caregiver.

Dr. Barry Jacobs offers three valuable suggestions in his book, *The*

Emotional Survival Guide for Caregivers. Dr. Jacobs' first recommendation instructs families to utilize the professional care available. Home health staff and nurse's aides can provide hands-on care and assist families in caregiving. The second way families can support their ill family member and primary caregiver is by sharing caregiving duties. Good communication will be enhanced by weekly or monthly conference calls or a family chat room. Family members can divide up the necessary chores and set up a caregiving calendar to schedule respite breaks for the primary caregivers. Family members might set up an account and make monthly payments to pay for support services for their parent.[39]

Dr. Jacobs comments that caregivers "have to be willing to use the available supports. That brings us to the third common problem of many family members caring for loved ones. They don't take full advantage of the help they're offered."[40]

Out-of-Town Family Members

Out-of-town caregivers can experience the same emotions as local caregivers and they also may deal with added stress and guilt because they're far away. When John's father suffered from a stroke, John paced the floor and worried about how to care for his parents who live 800 miles away. What should he do? Should he move his parents closer? If his parents don't want to move, where do they get reliable help?

The AARP experts give this advice to long-distance caregivers: discuss with parents (and other family members) what help they need and will accept. The parents may not want to move and leave their home and friends behind.[41] Using the Internet and telephone, long-distance caregivers can find community services their parents will find helpful and acceptable. Eldercare Locator at 1-800-677-1116 will refer caregivers to the Area Agency on Aging in each community.

Caregivers should recognize the social group their parents may belong to. Ask who you can call on when you need help. Caregivers should make a list of these friends, neighbors, clergy and extended family members with phone numbers, e-mail addresses and home addresses. Can any people on this list provide transportation or help with shopping or other chores? Who can be hired to mow Dad's grass?

If possible, a long-distance caregiver should work with his parents to get organized before a crisis occurs. Gather information such as illnesses, an up-to-date list of medications, and doctors' names and phone numbers.

A listing of Dad's financial information will simplify helping when Dad can't get to the bank. This information can include assets and debts, monthly income and expenses, a statement of net worth, and information on bank accounts, financial holdings and credit cards. Legal documents include wills or trusts, advance directives and powers of attorney. It's very important that caregivers know where to locate important documents (birth certificates, deed to home, insurance policies), Social Security numbers and information on health insurance and driver's licenses.[42]

Some caregivers will find their parents have purchased long-term care insurance. This insurance will help pay for in-home services or nursing home facilities, whichever is needed. Family members should learn the details of the long-term care insurance to best utilize the benefits of their parents' insurance plan.

The experts recommend talking to parents and deciding what they need and who can provide assistance. Will in-home housekeeping be sufficient help? Who can mow their grass and care for flowers? Parents may find it painful accepting help and be reluctant to make changes. If the parents recognize that assistance will help them continue an independent life, they may be willing to accept the assistance. Some parents will need financial help to afford services, and caregivers able to offer financial assistance can help in this manner.

How can out-of-towners support their caregiving siblings? Out-of-town siblings can provide tremendous support to the caregiver by listening in a nonjudgmental manner. They can take on specific tasks. Adult children can purchase clothing and shoes for Mom when they visit. Out-of-town siblings can check on Mom by phone calls and e-mails. They can access needed information by utilizing reputable organizations and services via the Internet. They may choose to pay for needed services such as lawn care or home health aides, or they can come stay with Dad for a week so the caregiver can relax on vacation.

Extended family can provide support and caring. When her cousins came to visit her and her mother, Ellen felt a sweet reprieve from her caregiving duties. She noticed her mother didn't complain as much as she enjoyed the attention of her niece and two nephews. Old family pictures were pulled out and Ellen's mom identified people in the pictures and reminisced about happier times. Ellen enjoyed the weekend reprieve a great deal. She was touched by the caring and attention her cousins showed both her and her mother. The cousins stayed at a nearby hotel and didn't cause any extra work for her. In fact, the weekend visit lightened her load as she realized that their extended family cared about them.

Sibling rivalries and painful memories can cause additional stresses during caregiving times. A family meeting can be an effective method to organize the families' resources. The Family Caregiver Alliance (FCA) suggests these guidelines: "set an agenda for the meeting and keep to it, focus on the 'here and now' ... share feelings with siblings instead of making accusations, listen and respect the opinions of all participants."[43]

The FCA recommends that the primary caregivers contribute to a positive situation by communicating on a regular basis the parent's condition and planned care. The caregiver should show siblings their help is wanted and needed by discussing problems and listening to their opinions. A sibling may offer an excellent solution that the caregiver hasn't considered. The caregiver should be willing to compromise. Utilize the knowledge and strengths of family members. The lawyer daughter can help set up a durable power of attorney for healthcare and bring Dad's will up to date. The nurse son can provide guidance when Mom needs medical care.

Each caregiver must recognize his own needs and care for self while he provides care for his loved ones.

4

Stress Breakers

Bob and Jan Gile included a mother-in-law suite in the plans for their new house. No one knew that before the house was finished they would be bringing Katie, Jan's recently widowed mother, to live with them. When her husband of 62 years died from pneumonia, Katie did not want to return to their home. Fortunately, a loving daughter and son-in-law had planned ahead. With a positive attitude, Bob and Jan moved Katie into their home and she flourished in that environment.

Attitude

The person who chooses to give or oversee care will do well to begin with a good attitude. The person who feels trapped into the caregiving roll begins with a problem.

A person may find that previous experiences with caregiving gives knowledge but also stressful memories. One woman had spent three years caring for her first husband until his death from a neuromuscular disease. When her aging parent required help in the parent's last years, she struggled with the obligation. While she loved her dad and wanted to be a good daughter and care for him, she found herself stressed as he required more help. After their father's death, she was talking to her big sister about what she called her own "bad attitude." Her sister pointed out how the earlier caregiving had affected her. Voltaire said, "Life is thickly sown with thorns, and I know no other remedy than to pass quickly through them. The longer we dwell on our misfortunes, the greater is their power to harm us."[1]

When a person tries to control a situation he cannot control, stress can occur. The experts at AARP say it this way: "Step back and accept it. You are not in charge of life. You won't be the perfect caregiver. You cannot handle every detail. You can't cure your parent's illnesses. You won't be able to change other people's personalities, their ingrained habits, their fixed prejudices. You are not going to become a saint who forgives all old wrongs and never speaks a harsh word. And that's okay. Just do what you can reasonably manage and accept that the rest of life, for better or worse, is going to flow past you. It really isn't up to you to make it all better."[2]

Live Today as It Comes

People who need to know what's coming next will find the future is often uncertain. When dealing with ill family members not even the doctors can accurately predict how and when certain events will occur. A schedule can be thrown askew by a sudden fever or illness in the family member. Experienced caregivers would recommend that a caregiver live each day as it comes. This healthy attitude recognizes that caregivers cannot control many aspects of their situation. Caregivers who adopt an attitude to live each day will find life less stressful and more pleasurable.

Enjoy the Small Pleasures of Life

Wise caregivers look for peaceful, relaxing times. It's often easier to scurry around in a cleaning frenzy than it is to sit quietly with the ill family member. Offering such companionship may initially be uncomfortable or may feel like a waste of time, but the sharing of quiet moments can benefit both the patient and caregiver.

Cherish Sweet Moments

Raymond loved to tell stories of the "good old days." He was raised on a farm in Kentucky until his family moved to Missouri when he was eight years old. Raymond always had to work hard. He told great stories of riding his horse to school, and later driving his first Model T Ford. He survived the Great Depression by working rented farmland (he couldn't afford his own). By hard work and perseverance, he provided for his family through good times and bad. Through example and sharing family history, he instilled in his children and grandchildren a good work ethic. Even in the weeks prior to his death at age 92, Raymond would get a faraway look in his eye as he shared his stories with family. Later his daughters would smile as they remembered how he enjoyed sharing stories.

Physical Stress-Breakers

Deep Breathing and Relaxation Exercises

Pain, anger and fear, all negative emotions, cause a person to take short, shallow, quick breaths. Positive emotions such as love, pleasure and relaxation cause a person to take long, deep breaths. A person can control his breathing to achieve a relaxed state.

Relaxation and deep breathing exercises help in coping with stress, anger, fear, and pain. Deep-breathing techniques can be used to "turn off the fight-or-flight response, lower blood pressure, ease panic attacks and control pain."[3] In fact, Harvard University researchers found that a person breathing slowly and deeply from the abdomen experiences increased blood flow to the brain and a 65 percent reduction in stress.[4]

How does one breathe with the abdomen? People usually breathe only from their upper chest. To practice deep breathing, find a comfortable place to lie down or sit. Place one hand on the stomach area below the breast bone, and notice whether that hand moves when breathing occurs. Take several deep breaths inhaling and exhaling. Does your hand move? Next, move that hand to the abdomen (below waist level). Practice taking a few deep breaths and notice whether the abdomen and the hand over it moves. Both should move as the deep breaths fill the lungs and move the abdominal area. Count to three while blowing out the breaths slowly. You can think of your abdomen as a balloon which fills with air as you breathe in. As you exhale, you can let your abdomen relax toward your spine.[5]

A word of caution: "After a few minutes, allow your breathing to return to normal. Don't keep taking deep, big breaths, or you'll make yourself dizzy.... If you feel dizzy or lightheaded, stop and return to your normal breathing until the feeling passes.... You may be a bit light-headed when you finish, so move carefully at first."[6] A person should rise slowly, orient himself, and be careful to keep his balance after deep-breathing and relaxing exercises. Deep breathing can be combined with meditation, visualization, yoga and other relaxation techniques.

Add Progressive Muscle Relaxation

Progressive muscle relaxation combined with deep breathing exercises also decrease muscular tension and stress. As a person breathes in deeply, he can tense a group of muscles and relax those muscles when exhaling. An audiotape may be a helpful guide while learning progressive muscle relaxation.

If possible, a person should lie on his back and stretch comfortably. One routine recommended by the Arthritis Foundation begins with the right foot, which is tensed (not to the point of pain) for three or four seconds, followed by exhaling and releasing all tension. Next the right knee and thigh muscles are tensed for three or four seconds and relaxed. By working one leg, then the other leg, the muscular tension and relaxation moves up the body and involves all major muscle groups. The continued tensing and relaxing of muscles includes the face as a person opens mouth and eyes comfortably wide, sticks out his tongue, and then relaxes his muscles. An all-over muscle tensing can be done, followed by a relaxing and quiet time of rest.

A word of caution from the Arthritis Foundation: "Tensing muscles that haven't been used much may bring on cramps or pain at first.... Tighten your muscles just enough to be aware of the tension. Awareness is the important point, not how hard you squeeze your muscles.... Breathing exercises may make you lightheaded until you get the hang of it, and deep relaxation may also make you a bit wobbly at first. So take a minute when you finish the exercises to reorient yourself. Get up slowly, being careful to check your balance."[7]

Hydrotherapy: A Warm Soak in a Tub

Sitting in a tub of warm (temps between 100 and 102 degrees Fahrenheit) water can be a quiet retreat from the stresses of caregiving. Add scented bath bubbles, soothing music and aromatherapy candles for a relaxing spa-like retreat. Warm water can calm while relaxing muscles and soothing sore, achy joints.

Researchers at the University of Minnesota included 40 healthy adults in a study looking at whirlpool baths versus warm baths. They found both whirlpools and warm baths produced "increased feelings of well-being and decreased state of anxiety. Whirlpool immersion decreased stress reaction though the tub did not."[8] Use caution to prevent falls because a warm bath often makes one sleepy and relaxed.

Exercise

Exercise, both aerobic and anaerobic, are effective stress management tactics. Mindful exercise such as yoga and tai chi are proven stress relievers. A busy caregiver may feel there's no time for exercise or they may feel guilty about taking time for self. During stressful times, caregivers must remind themselves that caregiving is a marathon: "Marathoners get through a race by pacing themselves and getting sustenance and water along the way."[9]

Walking

Walking decreases stress, anxiety and depression because the body releases its natural painkilling endorphins. A person's heart and lungs become more efficient when that person walks; LDL (bad) cholesterol is lowered and HDL (good) cholesterol is raised. Walking makes one's bones stronger, reducing the risk of osteoporosis, and muscles become stronger through the exercise of walking.

Walking is gentle to joints and costs only the price of a good pair of shoes. How does one pick out a good walking shoe? The *Arthritis Today Walking Guide* recommends that a person buy shoes where salespeople are trained to help fit shoes. Shoes should fit so that heels don't slide and the person's toes have room to spread out. A thumb's width between the end of the big toe and the end of the shoe is considered a proper fit. The soles of shoes should provide good traction on the walking surface: "Avoid sticky, non-skid soles and heavy rubber lugs, the part that curls over the top of the toe area; these tend to cause trips and falls. Likewise, avoid slick, smooth-soled shoes, because they make slips and falls more likely."[10]

Walking shoes should flex and bend at the forefoot while remaining fairly rigid through the midsole. An angled heel gives a rolling motion to each stride and helps prevent shin splints, tenderness and pain. A breathable fabric shoe helps keep feet dry. When the heel portion of the shoe is well cushioned, the shoe better absorbs the impact of each step. A good arch and heel support helps protects the walker's foot. The shoe closure can be personal preference, whether shoestrings or Velcro. Shoes should be replaced when they are worn out. "A walker who takes 30-minute walks three times a week might need replacements after about 9 to 12 months."[11]

A walker should wear comfortable clothes. Layering clothes allows a person to take off or put on items of clothing as needed to stay comfortable. Three layers are recommended for walking on a cold day: an inner layer of soft, lightweight, synthetic long underwear that dries easily, a middle layer of fleece or wool, and an outside layer which is water-resistant but vented to keep the walker warm and dry. A person preparing to walk also needs a hat, gloves and socks which wick away moisture.

Before beginning a walking program, check with your doctor for recommendations, especially if you have heart disease, are overweight or haven't been physically active. Begin walking slowly, warming muscles and allowing the heart to respond gradually. Then do some stretches and flexibility exercises before resuming walking at a quicker pace. The beginning walker should start slowly and gradually increase speed and distance: "A good pace is one at which you can still hold a conversation without too much huffing and puffing."[12]

Good posture helps protect joints. Look out ahead and watch for obstructions, potholes, and curbs to avoid falling. A cool-down, slower, pace for the last five minutes of the walk is recommended. You overdid the walk if you're exhausted when you finish. If you are still sore two hours after you walked, you overdid the exercise. Slow down and do less for the next outing and gradually build endurance. Safety is crucial. Watch for traffic. If no sidewalk is available, walk facing the traffic. If you walk at dusk or after dark, wear clothing which reflects lights and enables drivers to see you.

Massage

As Elaine enters a dimly lit room, soft music plays quietly. She disrobes and lies on her stomach, snuggling under the warm sheet and blanket as she answers the knock on the door: "Come in." The masseuse enters, speaking quietly, and begins the massage. For the next hour, Elaine lies on the massage table and progressively relaxes as her muscles are rubbed and oiled. When the massage is completed, she finds she can barely walk she's so relaxed. When she later describes it to her husband, he is surprised that she said her favorite places to have rubbed were her feet and the back of her neck into her hair.

Although massage is definitely relaxing, it's also beneficial. Researchers believe massage helps "boost immune system strength by increasing the activity level of the body's natural 'killer T cells' which fight off tumors and viruses."[13] Another benefit of massage therapy is the stimulation of endorphin (the body's own opiate, or painkiller) production in the brain. Massage therapy helps control pain in the following conditions: low back pain, breast and other types of cancer, after surgery, and migraine headaches. Studies show that massage therapy decreases anxiety and depression. Even a ten to fifteen minute massage has benefits of lowering a person's blood pressure and cortisol level, a stress hormone.[14]

According to the American Massage Therapy Association, the four most common types of massage include Swedish, deep tissue, sports and chair massage. Swedish massage involves rubbing or kneading the soft tissues of the body while warm oil is applied and rubbed into the skin. Deep tissue massage relieves tension in deep muscles and connective tissue of the body: "Often the strokes go across the grain of the muscles and the therapist will use fingers, thumbs and even elbows."[15] Sports massage "helps prevent athletic injury, keep the body flexible and heal the body should injury occur."[16] Chair massage involves the person sitting in a chair, fully clothed while the masseuse rubs the upper body, especially the shoulders and neck.

Gardening

For the practical-minded person, a garden means vine-ripened tomatoes and bell peppers, necessary ingredients for homemade salsa. For others, a garden means daylilies bursting with yellow sunshine and red roses on the stem. Whether it's vegetables, herbs or flowers, many people find gardening enjoyable. One can forget about problems and relax while digging in the soil and watering seedlings.

Researchers wondered how much exercise a gardener would get working in the garden. A small Kansas State University study involved 14 healthy gardeners (five women and nine men between the ages of 63 and 86). They found that gardening provided a moderate intensity of exercise. A significant finding was the amount of time these gardeners spent working in their garden: 33 hours a week during the month of May and 15 hours a week during June and July. The researchers concluded that gardening definitely meets the criteria of being an exercise and contributes to a person's physical and mental well-being.[17]

Common sense tips for gardeners include these: "put safety first ... watch out for heat-related illness ... know your limits ... enjoy the benefits of physical activity, get vaccinated (to protect from tetanus) ... and go green." A tetanus booster is recommended for most individuals every ten years.[18]

Tai Chi Chuan

Tai chi involves slow fluid movements and meditation to balance a person's vital life force, called "qi" (pronounced chee and sometimes spelled "chi" by Westerners). This 600-year-old practice is a vital part of traditional Chinese medicine, which teaches that disease results from blocks or imbalances in the flow of qi through the body. By practicing tai chi, a person can correct the blockages and imbalances of qi and achieve better health.

Tai chi, with its gentle, controlled movements and meditation, is recommended by many rheumatologists and doctors who believe it's good exercise for people with arthritis and muscle diseases. The gentle movements of tai chi strengthen muscles and improve balance while relieving stress and depression.[19] Experts recommend taking a class to learn tai chi. To participate, a person should wear comfortable, loose clothing and thin-soled shoes or go barefoot. Classes begin with a warm-up and deep breathing or meditation to quiet the mind followed by slow, graceful movements with poetic names such as "wave hands in clouds."

A word of caution: find a reputable health center with tai chi classes and don't overexert while doing tai chi. Tai chi is "soft and meditative; and should not be taught as martial arts. Ask the teacher about the goals of the class. If the class focuses on self-defense or hard, violent movements, it is not tai chi."[20]

Yoga

"Seated cobra" and "eagle pose" are the descriptive names of two yoga poses. Yoga is part of an ancient Indian healing system called Ayurveda. Yoga combines physical exercise, the mental aspect of meditation in an effort to bring body, mind and spirit into harmony. When practiced daily, yoga can improve flexibility, increase muscle strength, and decrease stress levels.

Talk to your doctor before beginning to verify that you are healthy enough to perform yoga. Take yoga instruction from an experienced teacher. Once the basics are learned in class, you can practice at home. Several styles are available. Watch a class to verify whether you like this style and whether it's an appropriate activity level. Wear comfortable, loose-fitting clothes. The postures are done barefoot on a nonslip mat or rug.[21] Experts recommend that each person purchase their own yoga mat and not share with anyone else to avoid the risk of foot infections, including athlete's foot.

Emotional and Social Stress Breakers

Avoid Isolation

Men and women react to stress differently. The experts at WebMD offer guidelines on how women can constructively deal with stress: have a support system of family and friends who are supportive and helpful in tough times, and find a friend who respects a woman's privacy and can keep a secret if needed. A woman should say "no" to more projects when she recognizes that she's stressed, and say "yes" to times of relaxation. Recommended stress management for a man includes exercise, spending time with the guys, solitary stress-reducing activities, and a support group of people who are trustworthy and care about him.[22]

Social support strengthens and renews a person. Sometimes the caregiver just needs someone to listen and empathize. Just being able to "vent" gives tremendous relief. Support groups, both formal groups and online groups, can help caregivers. During the support group meetings, people can share feelings and vent to others who listen. The caregiver will discover he isn't alone and will be able to cope better with the caregiver challenges.

Humor

"Death and dying are not funny, but funny things do go on even when there is death and dying." Author and "jolly-tologist" Allen Klein tells how he used humor to survive the death of his 31-year-old bride. Insights he shares in his book *The Courage to Laugh* include the following: "Death itself is not funny. Things that happen around it are. Our only real weapon against death is humor. Those who work in the death-and-dying arena understand the need for humor; those who do not, may not. Some people will never see the humor/death connection. Most people don't want survivors to be morose after they die. You can laugh and cry at a loss. Both are appropriate. No matter how serious a situation is, humor can help us get through the day."[23]

What does humor give to caregivers? Researchers at Loma Linda University in California have found laughter lowers stress hormone levels and blood pressure. Laughter improves immune function when the body produces infection-fighting T-cells (lymphocytes), immunoglobulin A and gamma interferon, all components of a person's immune system. A belly laugh fills the lungs with oxygen and decreases muscle tension. Laughter triggers the release of endorphins, the body's natural painkillers, and promotes a sense of well-being.[24]

Humor gives hope and strengthens a person's ability to cope. Laughter helps distract one from the problems a person faces and gives a reprieve from the pain, sorrow or worry. "Humor helps us keep our balance when life throws us a curve-ball."[25] By giving some distance from the problems, laughter helps people keep their balance.

A study done by University of Maryland researchers found that "people who laughed the least were 40 percent more likely to suffer from heart disease than people who laughed most frequently."[26] Humor can be used to connect people. They can use humor to help them deal with the five stages of death and dying: denial, anger, bargaining, depression, and acceptance.[27]

Mr. Klein points out the negative side of humor: it's harmful if it hurts a person's feelings, is used to avoid the truth or causes misunderstandings. Someone recovering from surgery may find laughter to be physically painful. He recommends that people use humor with a sensitive and caring attitude.

Journaling

Many journals written in difficult times have been turned into books by their writers. Journaling can be soothing to the writer. "It requires an absorbed concentration, an inner clarifying of feelings and thoughts, and a weighing and measuring of words that can induce a creative reverie."[28] Journaling requires the writer to step back and observe what's happening and how loved ones are being affected by the events.

A study by North Dakota State University asked people dealing with chronic ailments, specifically arthritis and asthma, to spend one hour per week writing about their lives. Forty-seven percent of the participants reported their symptoms improved in the weeks and months after they began journaling.[29]

Music

"A song is so much more than sound to us. It is a feeling, a memory, a new world, a trip back to an old world. Keep music in your life where you go." People ages 60 and older reported that listening to their favorite music helped improve their mood.[30] Since ancient times, music has been a part of promoting health in people. Over the centuries, medical people have recognized the benefit of music. Researchers find that music can reduce a person's stress under a variety of situations. Music before, during and after surgery speeds recovery while lowering the amount of pain medication needed and lowering cortisol (a stress hormone) release.

How does music affect the body? Many theories have been discussed. One highly regarded theory says that music is perceived in the right side of the brain but the left side may be involved also in analyzing music. The temporal lobe (where the ear and hearing are located) becomes involved and sends signals to deeper structures such as the thalamus, mid-brain, pons, medulla and hypothalamus. Through these deep structures, neurohormones and the regulation of adrenalin (epinephrine) occur, which affects the body.

The music which best decreases stress should please the listener. Some recommend Celtic or Native American songs as relaxing. Other people find sounds of nature tapes relaxing. Each person should decide which music he finds relaxing. For stress reduction, experts recommend music with "a tempo of eighty beats or less, slow flowing rhythms, a low, pitch, and repetition and placed at a moderate volume."[31] The listener can start with music that matches his emotional state and then gradually move to a slower, more relaxed music. Anyone can utilize music therapy to decrease his stress level.

Pet Therapy

Ginger, a blond Shih Tzu, was the best listener. She would turn her head to the side and sit quietly. She never interrupted. She shared the happy times and gave great puppy dog kisses when her people cried.

Caregivers who do not own pets probably would not want one more responsibility, the care of a dog or a cat. However, caregivers who are pet owners should recognize the benefits their animal brings to their health. Pets reduce stress for their family members. One National Institutes of Health (NIH) study involved 421 heart attack victims. After a year, the dog owners among the group "were significantly more likely to still be alive than were those who did not own dogs, regardless of the severity of the heart attack."[32]

According to the Centers for Disease Control (CDC), pets can decrease "blood pressure, cholesterol levels, triglyceride levels, and feelings of loneliness. Pets can increase your opportunities for exercise and outdoor activities, and opportunities for socialization."[33]

Each person should decide what type of pet they want, whether dog, cat, goldfish or other. When considering pet ownership, each person should consider their living space, lifestyle and preferences.

Visualization and Guided Imagery

Professional golfers practice visualization when they imagine that small white ball rolling across the green and dropping into the hole with a satisfying plop. A person wanting to relax might see himself lying on a beautiful sandy beach with the green-blue of the Caribbean lapping at his toes. As he recalls the sounds, smells, and images associated with his memories, he relaxes and relives a wonderful vacation. Using visualization or imagery, a person imagines what he wants to see happen. This technique can be used to control pain and decrease stress and anxiety. Many athletes use it to improve their athletic performance.

Guided imagery involves three principles: the mind-body connection, the altered state and a feeling of being in control. The mind-body connection says images created in the mind affect the body almost like they're real events. An altered state explains how a person can use guided imagery to heal better, block pain, and learn and perform better. The control principle says "when we have a sense of being in control, that, in and of itself, can help us to feel better and do better."[34]

Visualization techniques can be learned and practiced from a book or audio or classes. Classes can be found through stress management programs and mental health programs. If guided imagery allows nightmares or bad memories to surface, a person should get professional help.

Spiritual Stress-Breakers

Meditation, Prayer, and Spiritual Support

Meditation gained popularity in the mid–20th century. Meditation occurs when a person sits quietly and focuses his attention on an object, thought or sensation: "This can be a sound, a holy phrase, your own breathing or bodily sensations, or an image. In the West, prayer is the best-known meditation practice."[35] Research shows that meditation practiced on a regular basis relieves chronic pain and decreases anxiety. Time shortages plague family caregivers. Meditation and prayer can be practiced in small time frames. It's the quieting of the mind that reaps rewards of decreased anxiety and stress.

A caregiver would benefit from the companionship and support of a spiritual group. "Solitary spiritual practice may appeal to you, but studies suggest that it is the regular attendance at services that is good for your health."[36] People who retreat to a spiritual center find their souls nourished. Many organizations offer retreats which can refresh a person.

Friends Can Help

"The gifts we treasure most over the years are often small and simple. In easy times and in tough times, what seems to matter most is the way we show those nearest us that we've been listening to their needs, to their joys, and to their challenges."[37] Sometimes Jan and Bob's best friends bring supper (home cooked or takeout) and include Katie in the evening's visit. Other times Jan cooks a meal for them in their home. Including Katie in the evening allows for more frequent visiting, company for Katie and support for Bob and Jan.

A friend can help by listening in a nonjudgmental way. This can be the biggest gift a friend can give. Women tend to be more talkative and open in accepting emotional support than men. However, men and women can benefit from talks with an understanding listener. Sometimes the talks will involve problem solving, such as determining what resources are available to help Dad live at home. Other times the caregiver just needs a friend to whom he can vent and know that his complaints won't be repeated. During good times and bad, friends of caregivers can be there with caring hearts and listening ears.

Psychologist Barry Jacobs says "it's difficult to handle any level of sacrifice if you don't receive acknowledgement of what you're doing for your ill loved one, compassion for your plight, and endorsement of your reasons for doing what you're doing — for who you are instead of just what you do. The fact that many caregivers don't receive all three from their family members or neighbors is why they turn to support groups and counseling."[38] A sincere comment from a friend can make a caregiver's day: "I'm so proud of you and your sister. You both are doing such a good job caring for your mom. She's very content living in your home. You girls have gotten her new clothes and keep her hair fixed. You should be proud of how you're caring for her. I'm sure it's not always easy, but you're doing a great job."

Stay in Touch

Caregivers find out quickly which friends will follow through with help and support. Many people have good intentions but never follow through. Friends who truly intend to "be there" for their caregiver friends will make efforts. They will offer definite help, not vague offers: "Can I cook supper and bring it to you next weekend? What night would work for you? Let's discuss a menu." Another offer of help might be this: "I could come by after work one evening this week and sit with your mom for a couple of hours while you and John get out and have dinner, go to a movie or do whatever you want. I could do that either Monday or Thursday. Which is best for you?"

Live in the Moment — Be Mindful

"The secret of health for both mind and body is not to mourn for the past, worry about the future, or anticipate troubles, but to live in the present moment wisely and earnestly."[39]

A caregiver mom hurrying from a busy day at work may worry about what to cook for supper, what time Timmy's softball game starts, and whether she has time to stop by Dad's house to check on him. For this woman, living in the moment may seem irrelevant. She wishes she had more time or less to do. How can she possibly put more into her day?

This caregiver mom is living in the moment when she takes advantage of the red traffic light to take some big deep breaths, look at the blue sky and appreciate the quiet inside her car. She will be living in the moment at Timmy's softball game when she sits back, closes her eyes and listens to the sounds surrounding her. These quick respite breaks could help her cope with her busy life.

Many caregivers find they have regrets. They wish they had done more to help Dad. Or they wish they had done things differently. They believe their efforts weren't enough and blame themselves. To live in the moment, the caregivers should forgive self and not mourn for the past. Recognize that human beings aren't perfect and human efforts won't be perfect. Caregivers freed from regrets will be able to live wisely in the present.

Caregivers must care for self. Make it a priority and avoid the dangers of stress and becoming ill.

5

Looking Back Through History

Caregiving Throughout History

"Families have always taken care of their chronically ill or disabled loved ones. Neighbors helped neighbors if they did not have family around and communities even helped care for the ill among them; however, the nature of caregiving has changed drastically over the years."[1]

Writer Emily Abel in *Hearts of Wisdom: American Women Caring for Kin, 1850–1940* explains the caregiving duties involved "not just cooking, cleaning and assisting sick people with feeding and mobility but also delivering skilled medical care. Women dispensed herbal remedies, dressed wounds, bound broken bones, reattached severed fingers, cleaned bed sores, and removed bullets. The display of unusual healing abilities conferred honor and prestige on women in diverse locales and social strata."[2] Further, Abel says, "Caregiving dominated women's lives throughout the nineteenth century.... Because mutual aid was often a requirement of participating in social life as well as a form of insurance, responsibilities extended very broadly." Women worked together to care for people in their families, their community and the surrounding area: "Women in isolated rural areas sometimes cared for strangers who needed assistance far from home."[3] The caregiving duties of a community often involved women from different social backgrounds working together to provide for the ill and injured of their area. These women would share the responsibilities and take turns providing care, staying overnight when needed. Often there was no doctor close by, so any medical care fell to the community caregivers. Some women caregivers became gifted and knowledgeable healers. These women gained recognition among their neighbors and were the first to be called when care was needed.

Raymond told his family stories about the healing skills of his mother, Fanny Belle. He remembered that she made poultices and grew herbs which she used to treat sick family and neighbors. He recalled her riding sidesaddle on the horse, and as a child he rode behind her as they traveled to the neighboring farms where Fanny Belle treated the sick. This knowledge was taught to the next generation. "Girls learned to brew herbal remedies and prepared poultices the same way they learned other domestic skills — while helping their mothers at home and accompanying them on visits to ailing neighbors."[4]

Dr. John C. Gunn published a handbook in 1830 called *Gunn's Domestic Medicine, or Poor Man's Friend: In the Hours of Affliction, Pain, and Sickness*. This book, which gained such popularity that it required 19 separate printings over the next ten years, was considered the "chief home health aide" in the western United States (at that time Kentucky, Ohio and Tennessee).[5] *Gunn's Domestic Medicine* (dedicated to President Andrew Jackson) gave practical advice to family and community caregivers. In it, a reader could find information on the recommended care for toothache, cholera, dysentery and childbirth, among other things. Commonly used herbs, remedies and treatments were included. One paragraph discussed liverwort: "This plant grows so abundantly, and is so well known in the western country, that a description would be unnecessary. The excitement produced throughout the United States in consequence of its being a supposed remedy, or cure for consumption, led to a full investigation of its virtues, when like thousands of its predecessors, it has only proved to be an innocent palliative remedy. By using it as a tea, it assists expectoration, or a discharge from the lungs; allays the irritation of the cough; and in some instances, lessens the frequency of the hectic symptoms."[6]

Not everyone trusted doctors in the 19th century so they did not summon a doctor. Others called doctors when all their own efforts had failed and death appeared imminent. Even as recently at the early 1900s, when a doctor was available, he would visit the family home to treat the ill. But without inventions such as telephones and automobiles, calling a doctor required time and effort.

During the late 19th century and especially the 20th century, doctors began using scientific principles to make life better and safer for their patients, and they gained the trust and respect of the people. Hospitals became places of technology and healing. The focus moved away from the care given at home and community caregivers were utilized less. Caregiving became more a family situation. Today family members care for each other until hospitalization is needed for surgery or treatment and afterwards the patient returns home to recover.

Another reason caregiving has changed over the past century is because people are living longer and developing chronic diseases. The advances in medical care extend life. As has been mentioned, the average life expectancy for a baby born in 1900 was 46.3 years for a male and 48.3 years for a female. A baby born in 2005 has a life expectancy of 75.2 for male and 80.4 years for a female.[7] Modern-day families also deal with a mobile society where families relocate for jobs. This complicates the caregiving situation. When siblings live scattered out from New York to Los Angeles, the commute to visit Mom requires time and money.

Also, women work away from the home in larger numbers than in the past. In 1900 only 5.1 million professional women worked outside the home compared to 65.7 million in 2005. Experts project that 76 million professional women will be working by 2014.[8] Professional occupations include registered nurses, teachers, engineers, pharmacists, doctors, and lawyers.

These factors add up to the current situation: families struggling to care for their loved ones.

Medical History

In colonial America, medicine was more a trade than a profession. Few doctors were educated in a university, attended classes or heard lectures. Doctors were not licensed nor did they take tests to prove their knowledge and skill. In those days they were apprentice trained, learning from a practicing physician who taught them what he knew and did. "They titled themselves 'doctor' not because they had received a diploma, but for the simple reason that they were doing what men with university medical degrees usually did; they took care of patients."[9]

Back then no one knew about germs and viruses; no microscopes had been invented to enable researchers to see those tiny organisms which cause infection. It would be another century before Louis Pasteur saw organisms through a microscope and proved to the world that germs cause infection. The world of 1771 did not believe in germs or viruses, which makes the actions of a preacher named Cotton Mather and a young doctor, Zabdiel

Boylston, remarkable. They inoculated people for smallpox. Cotton Mather heard of the practice of inoculation from an African slave who had been inoculated as a child. Inoculation involved making a small cut on a person's skin and purposely infecting this open wound with drainage from a smallpox sore. The person would have a mild case of the disease and recover. Mather's interest in this topic was shared by Dr. Boylston.[10]

Smallpox has been eradicated because of the success of vaccination (a modern version of inoculation). Since ancient times smallpox was a very contagious, often fatal disease caused by a variola virus and spread through direct contact with bodily fluids or contaminated objects such as bedding and clothing. Symptoms of smallpox include high fever, malaise, head and body aches, and a rash which becomes pustules.[11] The colonial city of Boston was dealing with a smallpox epidemic when Cotton Mather and Dr. Boylston began by inoculating Dr. Boylston's son, Thomas, and two slaves, one an adult and one a boy. Fear was rampant and many in Boston were unhappy with the inoculation practice. Mather and Boylston were criticized, vilified and threatened. A grenade was thrown into Cotton Mather's home.

But the results proved the value of inoculation after the winter of 1721–1722. Of the 5980 Boston residents, 844 died from smallpox (14 percent death rate). Dr. Boylston had inoculated 244 people and only six of them died (2.5 percent death rate).[12] Dr. Boylston moved to London, where the Royal Society of London honored his efforts. He later returned to Boston to live out his life a wealthy celebrity.

American statesman Benjamin Franklin noted the success of inoculation and recommended it to George Washington, who decided the Continental Army troops would be inoculated in 1776 and 1777. This decision was called "one of the greatest strategic and medical decisions ever conceived by a wartime general,"[13] as Washington prevented a potential smallpox epidemic among his troops. Benjamin Franklin also recommended inoculation for both sessions of the Continental Congress in 1774 and 1775. Some attendees heeded the advice and others did not. At least one individual who refused to be inoculated succumbed to smallpox.

During the mid-eighteenth century efforts were made to improve medical education. Dr. John Morgan recommended university education and training for doctors. In 1760, officials in New York City passed a law saying no one could practice medicine or surgery without passing a test and obtaining a license. Wealthy American men who wanted to become doctors went to Europe, first England and later France, for formal education and training.

During the late 18th century and early 19th century an important influence on American medicine was Dr. Benjamin Rush. Doctors did not yet have the benefit of scientific knowledge of germ theory, human anatomy and physiology. Human dissection of cadavers wasn't acceptable practice in those days. Medical students learned the workings of the human body by studying charts and pictures which weren't accurate. In these times, acceptable care by physicians included bleeding, vomiting, blistering, and purging.

Bleeding involved a physician opening a vein and draining away blood: "Doctors bled some patients sixteen ounces a day up to fourteen days in succession (the average male human body contains one hundred seventy-five ounces of blood)."[14] Blistering involved placing an irritant such as mustard plaster on the skin to raise a blister. The fluid from the punctured blister was believed to be harmful matter leaving the body. Dr. Rush believed and taught these practices to many American doctors: "Armed with just a bleeding lancet, a few drugs, and various herbal and mineral concoctions, the country's ill-prepared and poorly educated doctors considered themselves competent to treat almost any condition."[15]

Over the years medical education went from apprentice-based to for-profit medical schools in the 1820s. These for-profit schools enabled more doctors to attend school but the schools might or might not provide a quality education to their students.

The late 19th century found well-to-do young American men traveling to Germany and Austria for medical training. The American medical establishment took a big step forward when the Johns Hopkins Hospital opened its doors in 1889. Four years later a medical school attached to Johns Hopkins Hospital was opened. Under the leadership of men like John Shaw Billings, William Stewart Halstead, and William Henry Welch, a university-based medical education and research-based medical practice became reality. "A Johns Hopkins medical education meant learning by doing.... No American medical school had ever provided a system that afforded appropriate education at all levels. It was a revolution in medical schooling of the first order."[16]

Through the late 19th century, many medical advances occurred. Anesthesia made surgery pain free. Aseptic procedures meant a person had a better chance of surviving a surgery and not dying from infection. Vaccines were developed for rabies, typhoid fever, diphtheria, and bubonic plague. X-ray technology was discovered by Wilhelm Conrad Roentgen in 1895; finally doctors could "see" a fractured bone.

Public health became a specialty in the late 1800s when Stephen Smith served as commissioner of the board of health of New York City. He began to clean up the city and set sanitation codes, codes needed because horse manure sat on the city's streets and flies swarmed to it; raw sewage ran down the street curbs and fouled the water supplies; dead animals were left where they died. Disease and decay were present in many of the nation's cities, not just New York City. When doctors advocated prevention of disease for the public, they gained favor in the eyes of people. Filtration of public water sources prevented disease. Pasteurization of milk killed germs and made milk safe. Fly control prevented typhoid fever. Hospitals for tuberculosis (TB) patients were opened.

The public learned of the scientific breakthroughs and technological advances being offered by doctors and hospitals. Doctors gained the trust of the public and the community caregivers were called on less and less. Various organizations within the medical establishment worked toward licensing examinations and establishing minimum standards of knowledge and skill by doctors, whether generalists or specialists.

During the early 1900s efforts continued that accomplished the closing of inferior medical schools. Leaders in these efforts used the Johns Hopkins Medical School as their quality model. They believed medical students should learn the sciences of biology, microbiology, pathology and physiology during their education and should also gain experience with hands-on care of patients. These efforts to provide a quality medical education resulted in the closing of many medical schools. By 1930, there were sixty-six medical schools in America.[17]

The 20th century brought amazing medical advances. During the first fifty years of this century advances included development of vaccines for diphtheria, whooping cough, tuberculosis, tetanus, yellow fever, typhus and influenza. In 1913 the electrocardiogram (EKG) was developed by Dr. Paul Dudley White. Edward Mellanby found that rickets is caused by vitamin D deficiency and this vitamin was synthesized and made available to the public. Insulin was identified and made available for control of diabetes in 1922. Sir Alexander Fleming discovered penicillin in 1928. Blood typing was developed and the first blood bank was opened in 1937. In the early 1950s the first cardiac pacemaker was invented.

The second half of the twentieth century brought more medical advances. More vaccines were developed for diseases, such as polio, measles, mumps, rubella, chicken pox, pneumonia, meningitis, and hepatitis A and B. The first kidney transplant was performed in 1954. The first human heart transplant was performed in 1967. The mysteries of human DNA were unraveled. The first test-tube baby was born in 1978 and Dolly the sheep was cloned in 1996. The artificial kidney dialysis machine was introduced in 1985.[18]

Modern-day people have gained much quality and quantity of life from the findings of scientists and doctors. Medical news and research findings are reported on nightly newscasts telling people how to improve their health, and premier medical organizations provide information for the same reason.

Anesthesia

Modern-day man cannot imagine undergoing surgery awake and in pain. Prior to the discovery of anesthesia agents, "in those dark days, many patients approached surgery as though facing execution, an often appropriate assessment of uncontained risks, including pain, hemorrhage, shock, and postoperative infection."[19] Individuals needing surgery often got their affairs in order in case they died. By contrast, people of today experience pain-free surgical procedures with expectations of going home to recover.

The earliest anesthesia drugs were ether and nitrous oxide. Ether was first made centuries ago, possibly as early as the 8th century, by an Arabian philosopher, Jabir ibn Hayyam. A British scientist, Joseph Priestly, is credited with making the first nitrous oxide in 1773. Both these drugs had been used recreationally, hence the terms "ether frolics" and "laughing gas." American doctors and dentists such as Crawford W. Long, Humphrey Davy, and William T. Morton contributed to the acceptable use of ether and nitrous oxide for pain-free anesthesia.

"America's greatest contribution to 19th century medicine" happened on October 16, 1846, when William T. Morton, a dentist, administered ether to a patient and achieved a pain-free state. The surgeon, John Collins Warren, excised a vascular lesion from the patient's neck. The patient later told them he was aware of the surgery but felt no pain. Dr. Warren's famous quote to the audience was, "Gentlemen, this is no humbug."[20]

A British doctor, John Snow, began researching ether, chloroform and other anesthetic drugs. He developed a face mask for inhalation of anesthesia gases which is similar to modern face masks used to provide oxygen and anesthetic gases. Dr. Snow wrote books and shared his findings about anesthesia. He gave chloroform anesthesia to Queen Victoria for the births of her last two children. Dr. Snow is called "the first anesthesiologist."

The "31½ Miles Long" slogan by dentist Gardner Q. Colton advertised pain-free tooth extractions. In 1869 Dr. Colton touted a scroll with the names of 55,000 patients who felt no pain when he pulled their teeth. He asked each patient to sign his scroll and claimed that 55,000 patients marching past in single file "would extend for 31½ miles."[21]

"Physicians of 60 years ago who practiced anesthesia with just a "rag and bottle" would be amazed to observe modern techniques in which fresh gas flows are metered precisely."[22] The first anesthesia techniques literally involved dripping ether onto a cloth held to the person's nose. There was no anesthesia equipment. Equipment was developed by doctors such as Dennis Jackson, Ralph Waters and Brian Sword, who invented the carbon dioxide absorber anesthesia machine. The copper kettle vaporizer developed by Lucien Morris allowed safer, accurate anesthesia dosages. By 1900, first generation anesthesia machines were being used in operating rooms. Many improvements and modifications have resulted in the anesthesia machines used in today's operating rooms.

Efforts to monitor a patient's vital functions became easier when blood pressure monitoring was proposed by George W. Crile and Harvey Cushing in 1902. Through the work of Thomas Lewis, James Herrick and Harold Pardee, electrocardiography was developed: "EKG (electrocardiogram) monitoring wasn't routinely used until after World War II due to the risk of explosive anesthesia gases and the cathode ray oscilloscopes."[23]

Regional anesthesia techniques were being developed also. Regional anesthesia involves blocking nerve sensation to specific areas of the body and for a specific time frame. These procedures include spinals, epidurals, and nerve blocks of extremities. Many modern mothers-to-be enjoy the epidural experience. These moms can be awake and able to participate in the births of their babies while experiencing no pain.

Anesthesiology as a profession can thank Francis Hoefer McMechan for his contribution of a professional journal, *Current Researches in Anesthesia and Analgesia*, the profession's oldest journal. Dr. Ralph M. Waters contributed to the development of academic training for anesthesiologists.

Modern day anesthesiologists (MDA) and certified registered nurse anesthetists (CRNA) can thank many doctors and dentists for their contributions. Today anesthesia is a highly respected and trusted profession with excellent outcomes for patients, who can expect pain-free surgery and a safe return home to recuperate from their procedure.

Germ Theory and Antisepsis

Hippocrates (460–370 B.C.) is often called the "father of medicine" and he believed pus was a bad thing. He recommended managing wounds by cleaning wounds with wine, bandaging, and then pouring wine on the bandage. Another important ancient surgeon and scholar, Galen (A.D. 130–200), disagreed. He believed that pus was essential to wound healing, calling it "laudable pus." This inaccuracy was passed down through centuries of medical teaching until the germ theory was promulgated.

The development of the microscope was a result of the efforts of several people. The glass lens was developed in 1268 by Roger Bacon. Over the centuries, Hans Lippershy and Galileo Galilei made contributions when they created telescopes. In 1597 Zacharias Jannssen and his son Hans recognized that a specific arrangement of glass lenses would enable them to see objects they could not see previously. In the 17th century an English scientist, Robert Hooke, and a Dutch microscope maker, Antoni van Leeuwenhoek, improved the microscope. Leeuwenhoek developed a microscope lens with a magnification of 270x, a big improvement over prior microscopes with their magnification of 20–30x. He used the microscope to recognize and describe protozoa and bacteria. Robert Hooke, the English father of microscopy, published a book, *Micrographia*, showing his observations, including plant cells.[24]

Louis Pasteur discovered germs while looking through a microscope searching for an answer to why a beer manufacturer's vats of beer were turning sour and being ruined. The idea that an organism too tiny to be seen without a microscope was causing putrefaction in beer and infection in humans was radical and not accepted at first. In the middle 19th century Pasteur worked with other scientists such as Robert Koch to develop vaccines for cholera in chickens, anthrax in sheep and rabies in humans.[25]

This quote explains the state of affairs before Joseph Lister's practice of antiseptic surgery was introduced: "The man laid on the operating-table in one of our surgical hospitals is exposed to more chances of death than the English soldier on the field of Waterloo."[26] As recently as the 1860s, patients undergoing major surgery in England died in large numbers. Almost half of the post-surgery patients died from infection.[27]

Joseph Lister introduced antiseptic surgery in 1867, applying to the operating room the knowledge Pasteur presented. He began to wash his hands often, and "using carbolic acid as an agent of antisepsis, he sterilized his instruments, soaked wound dressings, and sprayed the substance liberally around the operating area." His patients survived, although the caustic effects of carbolic — numb skin, cracked nails and sore lungs — soon caused Lister and others to abandon it in favor of other antiseptic agents."[28]

Alexander Fleming discovered penicillin in 1928. He saw the mold penicillium had contaminated a culture dish of staphylococcus. He noticed a halo ring around the staph germ and realized the mold had antibacterial power. Fleming found that this penicillin (as he named it) killed Gram-positive germs, including those which cause scarlet fever, pneumonia, diphtheria, and meningitis, and at least one Gram-negative germ.

Researchers Howard Florey and Ernst Chain would continue working on penicillin and started mass production of the antibiotic after the Pearl Harbor bombing of World War II so it was used to treat wounded allied soldiers.[29] Modern-day people benefit from the medical breakthroughs of germ theory and antisepsis developed by researchers such as Louis Pasteur, Joseph Lister and Alexander Fleming.

Development of Hospitals

In Colonial America "hospitals were few in number, poorly managed, and unable to provide administrative support to an affiliated medical school.... They were facilities of last resort ... no more than shelters for those who could not afford treatment at home, had no family to provide nursing needs, or lived in such adverse conditions that there was no space in their house for the sick or dying."[30]

"Few doctors worked out of offices or in hospitals in the nineteenth century." In 1873 only an estimated 2 percent of doctors had hospital privileges.[31] By the 1930s, five out of six doctors had hospital privileges. Few Americans used hospitals throughout the early years of this country. As late as 1873, "the nation had only 120 hospitals, most of which were custodial institutions serving the deserving poor. Middle class patients rarely entered hospitals."[32] By the early 1900s medical care had moved out of the family home and into the hospitals, which housed technologies such as laboratories where medical tests were run and radiology departments where X-rays were taken. By the 1940s the public felt that hospitals were the best place for a woman to have her baby. This resulted in the "increase of births in hospitals from 708,889 in 1931 to 1,670,599 in 1942."[33]

The 120 American hospitals of 1873 grew in quantity and quality. By comparison, a 2009 survey showed 5747 hospitals in the United States.[34] Efforts were made to make hospital patient care efficient with quality outcomes as early as 1910. Efficiency expert Frank Gilbreth used time and motion studies to encourage efficiency. Doctors such as Ernest Codman recommended standardizing hospital records and analyzing patient outcomes to show quality results. These ideas weren't always popular but efforts to improve efficiency and provide quality outcomes continue in present-day hospitals.

Nursing History

"Before the US Civil War, it was expected that women would be the primary caregivers in their homes and nurses were men who served in the military. During the Civil War, however, women were called upon to act as caregivers to the wounded because there were not enough male nurses to care for the mass casualties."[35]

In the days, months and years prior to the Civil War, people on both sides expected a war, if one came, to be over within a few months. No one planned for a four-year war fought on their own lands with civilians getting caught in the middle. Food stores ran short, and not enough guns and ammunition were available. The armories had to manufacture more weapons as the fighting dragged on. Soldiers had weapons such as rifle muskets, pistols and carbines and lead bullets called minié balls, which were more accurate and deadly than prior musket ammunition had been. Submarines and ironclad river and ocean vessels were used during the Civil War. Cannons caused a great deal of damage to soldiers on both sides of the war effort.

Medical care during the war was primitive. Not enough supplies were available and not enough surgeons or male nurses were there. "The death rate during the Civil War was astronomical with more than 620,000 deaths and 10 million cases of illness out of a population of 29 million. Two of every three people died from disease and infection. Deaths from dysentery and diarrhea were prevalent.... Surgeons did not know even to wash their instruments between amputations, so many patients died from massive infections."[36]

Into this tragedy stepped nurses such as Dorothea Dix, Clara Barton and Mary "Mother" Bickerdyke. Dorothea Dix began her work as superintendent of female nurses for the Union army during the Civil War, served throughout the war and received no pay. She worked to define what nurses could and should do, while setting a high standard for the nurses. Dix would not accept young, pretty women who wanted to get married. "She only accepted applicants who were plain looking and older than age 30. The nurses of Dix's day were bound by a dress code of modest black or brown skirts, and they could not wear hoops or jewelry."[37] Her work paved the way for the United States Army Nurses Corps, which became a reality during the Spanish-American War that began in 1898.

While giving care to soldiers, Clara Barton noticed the lack of supplies. She began collecting supplies and delivered them to battlefields from Bull Run to Fredericksburg and Antietam. Clara Barton's work paved the way for the American Red Cross.[38]

Mary (Mother) Bickerdyke was a 44-year-old widow who helped gather supplies from her local church members and took those supplies to soldiers at Cairo, Illinois. When she saw the sad conditions, she and Mary Safford began work organizing and improving the sanitary conditions in the Cairo hospital. She earned her nickname "Mother" from her young soldier patients. Through her efforts to improve the hospital and care of soldiers, Bickerdyke earned the respect of Union generals, including General Grant.[39]

Florence Nightingale, an English woman, became the model for American nurses. Born to a wealthy British family, Nightingale wanted to be a nurse. Her father encouraged her wishes to become an educated, professional woman. During the Crimean War, she went to a military hospital and found appalling conditions there: "Nightingale is best known for her working during this time. She and her band of nurses cleaned up the filthy, deplorable conditions in the hospital and prevented deaths from disease, dysentery, and infection."[40] She established nursing as an educated profession.

Wars always tax the resources of a country. They also provide an opportunity for doctors and nurses to learn. Soldiers suffer horrific injuries in large numbers, which gives the medical people plenty of opportunities to practice and learn. Wars have often created a shortage of medical people. As doctors and nurses volunteer to go to care for the injured soldiers, a shortage becomes apparent back home. Over the centuries the military has learned how to set up mobile medical facilities, providing emergency care to injured soldiers.

Modern-day nurses find they are members of a trusted, respected profession. In fact, the Gallup poll lists nurses as "consistently one of the highest rated professions in Gallup's annual honesty and ethics poll."[41]

Alzheimer's Disease

Say the word "Alzheimer's" and people become anxious. A German physician, Alois Alzheimer, first described this illness in 1906. Dr. Alzheimer's first introduction to "Frau Auguste D" occurred when her family brought the 51-year-old woman to his office. Frau Auguste D couldn't remember and believed her husband was being unfaithful. She also had difficulty speaking and comprehending what she was hearing others say to her. Over the next five years, Frau Auguste D's condition worsened and she died in 1906. With the family's permission, Dr. Alzheimer did an autopsy. He found a shrunken abnormal brain. There were fatty deposits in blood vessels, abnormal deposits in and around the brain cells and the brain cells themselves dead and dying. In 1910, this disease was named after the doctor who cared for Frau Auguste D, Dr. Alzheimer.[42]

In 1946 a nine-year-old boy fell off his bicycle and developed severe seizures. By age 16 this boy had experienced so many seizures, and such bad ones, that his doctor removed a part of his temporal lobe including the hypocampus area. The seizures were cured but the boy could no longer make new memories. From this boy's experience, doctors learned about the hypocampus area of the brain and that this small area of the temporal lobe is important for making new memories.

Through years of research, doctors recognized that Alzheimer's disease affects the hypocampus area of the brain and robs a person of the ability to remember recent events and make new memories. Through the 1960s little was known about Alzheimer's disease. Founded in 1979, the Alzheimer's Association became the premier medical association for research and support for people dealing with Alzheimer's Disease. The first drug the Food and Drug Administration approved for it was Cognex, in 1993. While progress is being made in understanding this illness, much remains to be done. Families still struggle with the disease, which steals the mental capacity of loved ones. Current information and research on Alzheimer's disease is available through the Alzheimer's Association at www.alz.org.

Cancer

Early medical writings — the Egyptian Ebers papyrus and the Smith papyrus — written around 1600 B.C. referred to cancer. The father of medicine, Hippocrates, coined the word "carcinoma" from a Greek word, *karkinoma*, meaning crab: "The claws of the crab symbolized a cancer's tentacles eating into flesh. The crab is still a common symbol for cancer."[43] Hippocrates believed human bodies contained four "humors" (body liquids) — blood, phlegm, black bile and yellow bile — and that an excess of black bile caused cancer.

Galen, another Greek physician, who lived more than 500 years later than Hippocrates (A.D. 150) built on Hippocrates' hypothesis that excess black bile caused cancer. Galen taught that cancer was a systemic (affecting the entire body) disease and should be treated with their current treatments plus diet and purging. Galen's teachings were valued for 1300 years, until the late Middle Ages. The first anatomy book, called *De Humani Corporis Fabrica* [*On the Construction of the Human Body*], was written in 1543 by Andreas Vesalius. Vesalius proved Galen's black bile theory wrong. An English doctor, William Harvey, performed autopsies and learned how blood circulated through the human body. He published *De Motu Cordis* [*On the Motion of the Heart*] in 1628. Over a century later, an Italian, Giovanni Morgagni, began to relate autopsy findings to the patient's illness. His work began the study of cancer (oncology).

Prior to the first successful anesthesia in 1846, few treatments were available. Afterwards, surgeons could perform surgery with the hope of curing the patient. Over the past century chemotherapy, radiation therapy, hormone therapy, immunotherapy and targeted therapies have been developed. "Cancer is the second leading cause of death in the United States. Half of all men and one-third of all women in the United States will develop cancer during their lifetimes.... The risk of developing most types of cancer can be reduced by changes in a person's lifestyle, for example, by quitting smoking and eating a better diet. The sooner a cancer is found and treatment begins, the better are the chances for living for many years."[44]

6

All Things Medical

Understanding doctors and nurses will be easier if a person recognizes they are people. They're smart people who went to school at considerable expense for many years to gain the knowledge they have. Most of them went to that effort because they want to help people stay healthy or recover their health if they're sick. Many of them spend years paying back the student loans they needed to finish their education. But they're still people — people with the same frailties and humanness that all people have.

The patient and family may get tired and impatient while waiting for the doctor to see them. However, they may not know that doctor has been awake since 3 A.M. caring for another patient. An all-too-common scenario might involve that doctor crawling out of his bed in the early hours to visit a patient who is having a heart attack and has arrived at the local emergency room. For this doctor, his schedule is thrown off balance and he may feel he's swimming through molasses as he tries to catch up on his schedule the rest of the day.

What are the different types of doctors? A medical doctor (MD) and doctor of osteopathy (DO) both spend a minimum of six to ten years in specialized training. While they are in school, doctors decide whether to be a family practice/primary care practitioner or another type of specialist.

Everyone needs a family practice/primary care doctor, who provides oversight of a person's health, giving advice and guidance on a regular basis. The family practitioner might say, "I see a mole on your left leg. It looks fine now but you should inspect it on a regular basis and let me know if you see any changes occurring" or "You have gained ten pounds over the last year and you should work on losing that weight." This doctor will write needed medication prescriptions when a person has bronchitis or any other medical condition.

Specialists include many other types of doctors. With the ever increasing amount of medical knowledge and information, specialists have become more available.

Surgeons perform surgery. There are many types of surgeons. Ophthalmologists (eye surgeons) perform cataract extractions. Some get special training to repair detached retinas. Orthopaedic (bone) surgeons perform total joint replacements, repair cut tendons and nerves and set broken bones so they heal correctly. Neurosurgeons perform craniotomies (brain surgery) to remove tumors and relieve the pressure when a hemorrhagic stroke (cerebral bleed) occurs. They can perform surgery on a person's spine relieving pain and adding stability with implants when needed. Oncology (cancer) surgeons are trained to perform surgery as a part of the cancer treatments. General surgeons perform laparoscopic cholecystectomy (removal of diseased gallbladders through tiny incisions) and repair hernias among many other procedures.

Medical doctor specialists such as rheumatologists (arthritis) and oncologists (cancer) and pulmonologists (lung) utilize medication to treat people. Radiologists interpret patients' X-ray films and scans. Pathologists examine tissue specimens removed during surgery or biopsy and identify disease. Trauma physicians care for people injured during an accident or assault and usually work in the emergency department and guide patient care.

Finding a Primary Care Doctor

The medical world can be confusing and intimidating. How can a caregiver find the help he needs? Start with a family practice/primary care physician who knows the patient and can help navigate the confusing medical world. "Studies show that people who have a regular doctor get better care and are likely to stay healthier than people who look for a doctor only when they're sick."[1] Check with the insurance company to find their approved list of doctors in order to protect a person's financial status. When a person sees a doctor on the "approved list" the insurance company will pay a higher percentage of the bill.

Senior citizens enrolled in the original Medicare coverage have unlimited choices in doctors, hospitals, and other providers. People signed up with a Medicare Advantage Plan (like an HMO or PPO) will need to choose doctors, hospitals and providers approved by that plan. If they don't use preferred providers, the patient and family will pay more or all of the costs.[2] Online information about Medicare, Medicare Advantage and Medicaid can be accessed at http://www.medicare.gov/Publications/Pubs/pdf/10050.pdf.

When seeking a doctor, begin by asking friends and family for their input. No one person can please everyone, but a caring, knowledgeable doctor will usually get good reviews. If you know a nurse or other medical personnel, that person can give his opinion on the question of which doctor he would take his mother or father to see.

A board certified doctor is considered better when compared with a doctor who is not board certified. Board certified physicians and surgeons spend extra time and money to prove their excellence. These board certified physicians and surgeons are evaluated for the highest level of education, ethics, surgical competency and professional qualifications. A board certified surgeon lists "FACS" after his name. "FACS" means that surgeon is a Fellow of the American College of Surgeons. Other specialties have different initials indicating their board certification status.

"Board eligible" surgeons haven't yet taken their national examinations. Dr. David Sherer makes this recommendation: "It's a good idea to find out if the surgeon is in practice with others who are already board certified. That tells you that other, more experienced hands are happy to have this surgeon on their team. They trust his or her work and have confidence that the doctor has the skills and knowledge to pass the board certification exam when the time comes."[3]

Internet Sources

Reputable doctor's organization Websites on the Internet can help in your search for a doctor. The Website of the American Medical Association (AMA), www.ama-assn.org, can be used by consumers searching for doctors by specialty or by name. The American Medical Association also provides information under its "Patient" section. For example, a person could gain understanding of the brain by studying the "Atlas of the Body" under the "Patient" section.

The American Board of Medical Specialties' Website, www.abms.org, provides information to "consumers" which includes a list of board certified physicians. The American College of Surgeons at www.facs.org provides patients and family access to a directory of board certified surgeons and a "patient resources" section with reliable health information. Anyone needing accurate information about a colostomy could begin his research at this Website.

How does one talk to a doctor? The American Academy of Family Physicians makes these suggestions: tell the doctor about current symptoms and pertinent health history: "There's a swollen, red spot on Mom's leg. It has gotten bigger and it feels hot. Before this spot became a problem, she had been doing ok. Here's the sack containing her medicines." Take the bag containing all current medications, including over-the-counter, vitamin and herbal supplements or a list of these medications. One should tell the doctor if medications seem to be causing a problem. An up-to-date history of immunizations should be included.

A person can utilize the personal health information document available in this book to keep track of his health information. When Tom cut his hand, he wondered how long it had been since he received his last tetanus shot. An up-to-date personal health information document can answer that question.

Doctors speak medical language and nonmedical people can easily get lost. "Don't be afraid to speak up. It's important for you to let your doctor know if you don't understand something."[4] Caregivers should come prepared by writing down pertinent questions before the appointment. Ask which staff member in the doctor's office will be accessible if questions arise. The doctor's office staff such as a physician assistant (PA) or nurse can be a valuable resource.

Other Resource People

Registered nurses (RN) can be found in hospitals, clinics and doctors' offices in every city and town. The Gallup poll has listed nurses as the most trusted profession for the past eight years (since 2001). Nurses "are trained to be patient educators and, when necessary, advocates."[5] When one must be in the hospital, the nurse is a valuable resource. The patient will find RNs working around the clock. These nurses often recognize problems in the patient's condition, alert the doctor and give appropriate nursing and medical treatments before a crisis happens. A person should talk to his nurse and ask questions about his health status, any medications and any treatments that are planned. If the nurse cannot answer them, she will alert the appropriate doctor to answer these questions.

While a person is in the hospital, nurses administer all needed medications whether it's chemotherapy, antibiotics, or pain medicine. Simple things like the noise level at night or being cold and needing extra blankets are within the nurse's or nursing assistant's domain. The nurses are the ones who "know how to deal with the day-to-day problems of hospital life."[6]

Advanced Practice Nurses (APN) are registered nurses with advanced training and knowledge. These nurses with master's and doctoral degrees function in jobs such as nurse midwife, nurse anesthetist, nurse educators, and nurse practitioners in several specialties, including family practice and pediatrics. They are licensed in the state where they work and may become certified through specialized tests. For example, certified nurse midwives (CNMs) and certified registered nurse anesthetists are two groups who become certified as advanced practice nurses.

Nurse practitioners are APNs who are increasingly assisting in patient care by doing duties previously done by doctors. NPs will often be found in family practice groups; they are trained and educated to perform checkups, take patient histories, prescribe treatments and medicines, and order diagnostic procedures and lab tests. NPs expand a physician's ability to handle his patient load by giving caring, quality care, to their patients.

Assisting the RNs are support people such as licensed vocational or practical nurses (LVNs or LPNs) and unlicensed assistive personnel (UAP). Both LVNs and LPNs graduate from a practical nursing program and are licensed by the state in which they work. UAPs may have attended a formal "nurses assistant" program or they may be trained on the job. Often nursing and medical school students function in the UAP role while working throughout their college years. "Many LPNs and UAPs are hard-working, caring individuals who assist the nurses in providing for the patient's needs."[7]

Dietitians and nutritionists can teach a newly diagnosed diabetic person how to manage diet for better control of blood sugar. This diabetic and his family might want to attend classes where a dietitian and a nurse teach cooking and meal planning, classes which would help them understand and apply the information they've received about diabetes.

A person will see therapists in hospitals such as occupational, physical, and respiratory therapists. Both occupational and physical therapists complete a master's or doctoral program in their specialty and are licensed by the state in which they work. Respiratory therapists complete either a two-year associate's degree or a four-year baccalaureate degree in their specialty before taking a national certification test. After passing this certification test, respiratory therapists are certified (CRT). They can complete two more national exams to become a registered respiratory therapist (RRT).

Occupational therapists (OTs) work to improve quality of life. A senior adult who wants to continue living at home would find a fall prevention program taught by an OT valuable. Occupational therapists teach classes and work with individuals and family planning adaptations to the environment in order to increase their independence, promote health, and prevent further injury or decline. The full spectrum of occupations should be considered, from ADL (activities of daily living such as dressing, bathing, and other self-care activities) to IADL (instrumental activities of daily living which includes meal preparation, clothing care and home maintenance) to play and/or leisure (playing cards, watching TV, reading a book, enjoying hobbies).[8]

Physical therapists (PTs) help people restore mobility. Physical therapists excel at working with people who have arthritis, back or knee pain, shoulder pain, overuse injuries, osteoporosis, stroke and other debilitating conditions. Physical therapists will teach a person how to properly use crutches while a broken ankle is healing. They teach a person recuperating from carpal tunnel surgery how to regain mobility and strength in the hand, and they work with a war veteran as he learns how to use a prosthetic leg.

Respiratory therapists help people who experience difficulty when breathing. People with chronic lung problems such as asthma, emphysema and bronchitis will be assisted with lung function therapy by respiratory therapists. If a patient has several ribs broken during an accident, the ability to breathe would be limited, they would probably be admitted into the intensive care unit where ventilator assistance can be given to support breathing until the fractures heal and breathing is adequate. Respiratory therapists would watch over the patient's status and ventilator equipment during this time.

Social workers can provide valuable guidance during a confusing time. When a caregiving recipient is hospitalized, caregiver family members can ask for a social worker consult. Social workers know the local resources available to that family and can direct a family to services they need for their loved one.

Everyone should consider the pharmacist a valuable asset, as pharmacists are the experts on all drugs, whether prescription, herbal or over-the-counter. Problems with polypharmacy (side effects and interactions which can occur when a person takes multiple medications) can be decreased by using the same pharmacy for all medications. Ask a pharmacist to look over a filled-out personal health information sheet and check the drugs for interactions.

Understanding the Illness

Psychologist Barry Jacobs says "not having basic knowledge about the patient's illness is like driving some pitch-black country road without headlights and being jolted by every dip and thrown by every curve. Without understanding the rigors of the terrain, you're hard-pressed to prepare yourself for the ride or even just whether you're up to the journey.... [I]t's essential to have at least a rough map of the illness's course so you can plan for the major landmarks and decision points on the road to recovery or demise."[9]

Caregivers can gather information about Dad's heart condition, beginning with the doctor's office as pamphlets and booklets are available there. Reputable health organizations such as the American Heart Association, the Alzheimer's Association, and the National Cancer Institute provide information online and in pamphlets. The American Academy of Family Practice Website is accessed at www.familydoctor.org.

Basic information about five major health topics is given beginning in chapter 11 in this book. The five health topics include Alzheimer's disease, arthritis, cancer, diabetes, and heart disease.

Health Care Advocate

During a loved one's hospital stay, caregivers may find themselves in the role of health care advocate for that loved one. A health care advocate is someone who is able and willing to look out for the loved one's best interest during a hospital stay. This person can be the power of attorney or guardian but does not have to be. If possible the person serving as health care advocate should be "medically knowledgeable ... assertive but not aggressive ... trustworthy ... available ... familiar with any special fears or concerns, wishes or instructions ... organized."[10]

Choosing a Hospital

Are all hospitals created equal? Apparently not. How does a person find the best hospitals? Begin by talking with one's primary care doctor, who can guide this decision. Even if this doctor is on staff at several hospitals, he may recommend Hospital A. He may say, "Because of your history of heart disease, the cardiologists and cardiac surgeon at Hospital A are top-notch. If I needed open heart surgery, hospital A would be where I would go."

Look for accreditation by the Joint Commission. The Joint Commission, formerly the Joint Commission on Accreditation of Healthcare Organizations, is a nonprofit organization dedicated to quality health care. They inspect and certify more than 19,000 health care organizations in the United States and worldwide. Online information about hospital accreditation can be accessed at www.qualitycheck.org. For travelers who want to access Joint Commission accredited facilities internationally, this information can be accessed at http://www.jointcommissioninternational.org/JCI-Accredited-Organizations/. Joint Commission accreditation means quality in health care.

Check insurance coverage to ensure the hospital chosen is on the insurance company's "preferred" list to achieve the best financial coverage. If a person wants to use a hospital outside the preferred list, he should be prepared to pay the larger portion of the bill that will result.

Look for announcements which show quality. Hospitals that achieve excellence will broadcast those results. "Best in Missouri for Total Joint Surgeries" and "Magnet Status for Nursing" are two examples of quality which hospitals want the public to hear. Look for large volumes in the specialty a person needs. Researchers have proven that a facility, surgeons and staff who perform specific surgeries day after day, week after week become very proficient. For example, a high-volume "total joint" hospital gives the best patient outcomes for total joint surgery. This facility may dedicate an area for the care of total joint patients. The surgeons and operating room staff achieve excellence in their skills and knowledge. The nurses and staff on the total joint postoperative unit know how to care for those patients: "They quickly spot potential problems, take appropriate nursing actions, and work with the surgeon for the patient's best outcome. The physical therapists have experience with total joint patients. The physicians and nursing staff are adept at dealing with the chronic health problems found among total joint patients."[11]

Ask for a tour of the facility. If a prospective patient calls the public relations department in most hospitals and asks for a tour, it usually will be granted. On the tour, notice whether the hospital looks clean and attractive. Does it smell good? Are the staff members friendly? Are the patient rooms attractive? Are they private rooms or semiprivate? Is the bathroom private? Is there room for a person's family members and healthcare advocate?

Hospital-Based Doctors

When a person goes to a hospital, there are doctors employed or contracted to work at that facility. These doctors include hospitalists, anesthesiologists, radiologists, and pathologists. The patient does not have to find these doctors; they're available through the hospital.

Hospitalists work only in hospitals and they're trained to "care for patients who are sicker and require more treatment than those your primary-care doctor sees in the office. Whenever you're in the hospital, there's a good chance that you'll have one of these physicians caring for you as your full-time in-hospital doctor or covering for your primary doctor."[12] After discharge, the patient will see his primary-care doctor just as before the hospitalization.

Medical Doctor Anesthesiologists (MDAs) are the experts of anesthesia and pain control during surgical procedures and childbirth. These specialty trained doctors do more than administer anesthesia; they look at the patient's health status in their efforts to make anesthesia safe: "In the preoperative, phase, they listen to the patient's lungs and heart, and check on lab tests and electrocardiogram results to ensure optimal results."[13] During the surgical procedure, MDAs can provide anesthesia or provide oversight and assistance to certified registered nurse anesthetists. Postoperatively, the MDAs check on each patient and provide orders for any needed antinausea drugs or pain medications. MDAs watch over each patient's overall anesthesia experience.

Radiologists oversee the radiology departments in hospitals. Radiologists interpret those black and white films called X-rays. They "read" CT scans and MRI scans, providing doctors and other hospital staff with interpretations of all radiology tests.

Pathologists look at human tissue to see whether it is cancerous or not. Their reports help guide the patient and the surgeon in deciding what treatments are needed. Pathologists oversee laboratories.

Know Your Rights as a Patient

Everyone has rights when they become a patient. See *Know Your Rights: A Speak Up* document from the Joint Commission found on page 91 in this book. When people know their rights and their role in their own healthcare, better results can happen. The same is true for caregivers: they should learn the rights of their loved one during a hospital stay.

Confidentiality and privacy regarding a person's health status and medical records gained a giant step when Congress passed the Health Insurance Portability and Accountability Act (HIPAA) in 2003: "HIPAA allows you to look at, request changes to, and get copies of any health-information document kept about you and your care."[14] HIPAA provides privacy because it limits by federal law access to a person's medical record.

Legal Documents Involving Medical Care

The two documents which involve medical care are the durable power of attorney for health care and a living will. A durable power of attorney for health care appoints someone to make decisions about a person's health care. For example, Suzanne appointed one of her daughters as her durable power of attorney for health care. After Suzanne was diagnosed with Alzheimer's, she became mentally incapacitated. At that time, Suzanne's family agreed she could no longer live at home and they moved her to a secure Alzheimer's unit. As Suzanne's health continued to decline, her family used the durable power of attorney for health care document to enroll her in hospice care at the Alzheimer's unit. Under the care of her family, the nursing home staff and hospice staff, Suzanne lived 10 months longer before quietly dying in her sleep. Her family was with her when she died.

A living will allows a person to state his wishes regarding life-prolonging procedures. Both durable power of attorney for health care documents and living will documents vary from state to state. Each state provides this document, often free of charge. An example of the Missouri document is included in this book on page 102.

The difficult part of making a living will and a durable power of attorney for health care may be making some tough decisions. For example, if Elaine was comatose with no chance of recovery, what would she want done? Would she want compassionate care until she died? Would she want a feeding tube when she could not eat? Would she want cardiopulmonary resuscitation (CPR) if her heart stopped beating? Every adult needs to make those decisions and write them down in a living will. Then they will know their wishes will be honored.

The second step is for Elaine to give copies of her living will/durable power of attorney to her doctors, lawyer, family members and health care advocate.[15] Hospital staff will ask about a living will/durable power of attorney when a patient is admitted to the facility.

Medicare Versus Medicaid — What's the Difference?

Original Medicare is the federally funded insurance plan which began in 1965. American citizens over age 65 are eligible. People under age 65 with disabilities may be eligible for Medicare coverage. Original Medicare Part A covers hospital inpatient services, hospice care and home health services. Original Medicare Part B covers doctors' office visits, outpatient care and some preventive care services. If a person wants prescription drug coverage under the original Medicare program, they must enroll and pay for Medicare Plan D. Medicare Part C covers the Medicare Advantage (MA) plans. People who choose to enroll in Medicare Advantage plans should know these plans are offered by private companies and approved by the Medicare program. Anyone interested in a Medicare Advantage plan should learn the details of coverage. Medicare Advantage plans provide Part A (all parts of plan A except hospice services) and Part B (medical insurance). Some MA plans cover prescription drugs. MA plans provide choices of coverage such as health maintenance organizations, preferred provider organizations, and private fee-for-service (PFFS) plans. Under those plans, the choices of doctors, hospitals and other providers may be limited. "Not all Medicare Advantage Plans work the same way, so before you join, find out the plan's rules, what your costs will be, and whether the plan will meet your needs."[16]

Medicare Part D — Prescription Drug Coverage

Medicare Part D is available to anyone who has Medicare Part A and B or Part C coverage. These drug plans vary in the drugs covered and how much the plans costs. A person wanting to enroll should begin by gathering all his prescription drugs (taken on a regular basis). Researching which plan could include accessing www.medicare.gov and selecting "Compare Drug and Health Plans," "Compare Medigap Policies" or "Coverage Gap Information." Enrollment in a Medicare drug plan can be accomplished in several different ways: by completing a paper application, calling the drug plan phone number, or calling 1-800-MEDICARE (1-800-633-4227).

Medicaid

Medicaid is a program funded from both federal and state sources which assist people who have limited resources and income. Medicaid varies from state to state, so details such as who is eligible, how to apply and benefits available may be different in each state. Begin the search for details of the Medicaid plan at http://www.cms.gov/home/medicaid.asp.

What Is Hospice?

Hospice services provide physical, emotional and spiritual care to a person and his family when a cure isn't possible and death is expected to occur in a matter of months. Hospice is a "concept of caring derived from medieval times, symbolizing a place where travelers, pilgrims and the sick, wounded or dying could find rest and comfort.... Hospice affirms life and regards dying as a normal process. Hospice neither hastens nor postpones death."[17] Hospice services emphasize quality of life, comfort and pain control while a person is terminally ill. A person may think hospice is only for people dealing with cancer, but people dealing with terminal illnesses such as heart disease, AIDS, Alzheimer's, pulmonary disease, and neurological disorders can qualify for hospice programs.

Hospice staff members include doctors, nurses, aides, social workers, counselors, spiritual caregivers and volunteers. These hospice workers give physical care and emotional and spiritual support to both the patient and the family, and they provide pain relief when a person with terminal cancer suffers pain. Hospice staff members offer bereavement support to the patient and family throughout the stay in hospice and after the patient's death.

Who qualifies for hospice services? A person qualifies for hospice when he is diagnosed as being terminally ill and has a projected life span of six months or less. Payment for hospice services can be obtained from Medicare coverage Part A for a person who has Medicare coverage.[18] Some health insurance companies pay for approved hospice coverage. Many states have a hospice program for Medicaid recipients. For a family who does not have insurance coverage to help pay for hospice, some hospice services provide services without charge to individuals who have limited resources.

Prescription Drugs

The top causes of death from disease in 1900 can now be cured, or at least treated, by prescription drugs. In 1900, mortality rates per 100,000 population were tuberculosis (201), influenza (flu) and pneumonia (181), heart disease (123), infant diarrhea and enteritis (108), diabetes (92), cancer (63), diphtheria (43), and typhoid and paratyphoid fever (39).[19] The infectious killers of the past aren't even listed in the top three causes of death in 2006, which are heart disease, cancer and stroke (cerebrovascular diseases). The miracle medicines called antibiotics have saved countless people's lives.

Prescription drugs have improved life span and quality of life for millions of people. They've cured infections and controlled many chronic illnesses like high blood pressure (hypertension) and diabetes. Prescription vaccines have made diseases like smallpox and typhoid rare occurrences. These drugs do tremendous good and Americans love their prescription drugs: "For almost every malady, real or imagined, there's probably at least one FDA-approved drug sitting in pharmacies and another barrelful in the pharmaceutical-industry pipeline on the way. Americans downed more pills and supplements every single day in 2005 than inhabitants of all developed countries gulped down in a month in 1950."[20]

Prescription drugs, even with all their positive benefits, can cause problems. Every drug has side effects. Even the old familiar stand-by drugs like aspirin and acetaminophen (Tylenol) can cause problems if used incorrectly or in too large a dose. Aspirin can increase the risk of bleeding. In toxic doses, acetaminophen can cause liver damage. Caregivers need to recognize that their loved one may face the danger of being overmedicated. A person's kidneys and liver act as filters which rid the body of waste products, including broken down, metabolized drugs. A healthy person's kidneys and liver cope with this work well. However, as a person ages, his kidneys and liver may struggle to filter the body's waste products and break down any prescription drugs he takes. For this person, the doctor may need to prescribe a lower dose of medication and may avoid prescribing some drugs altogether.

When multiple medications are taken, drug interactions are possible. This phenomenon is called polypharmacy. Polypharmacy means "many drugs." It has been defined as a person taking multiple drugs (including prescription, over-the-counter, and herbal) with resulting side effects and problems. People with chronic health problems often find they're seeing multiple doctors and receive multiple prescriptions. Also, adding over-the-counter medications to prescriptions can cause problems. For example, a person may be taking a prescription nonsteroidal anti-inflammatory for knee arthritis. When this person takes over-the-counter ibuprofen for a headache or fever, he may be taking too much of this type medicine.

What are the symptoms of polypharmacy? Sometimes symptoms begin after a person starts taking a new medicine. Sometimes symptoms begin gradually and take a while to become evident. Signs and symptoms of polypharmacy or side effects include "tiredness, sleeping or decreased alertness, constipation, diarrhea or incontinence, loss of appetite, confusion (all the time or only sometimes), falls, depression or lack of interest in usual activities, weakness, tremor, hallucinations (seeing or hearing things), anxiety or excitability, feeling dizzy, decreased sexual behavior, or skin rashes."[21]

How does a person and his caregiving family avoid harmful drug reactions? The American Geriatrics Society gives these recommendations: "Ask before taking an OTC (over-the-counter) ... make a list (of medicines including herbals and over-the-counter) ... share it (show this medication list to the doctor at every visit) ... ask questions (about new medicines or changes in a medicine) ... update (the drug list) ... read labels ... follow directions ... try to use one pharmacy for all prescriptions ... review and revise (the medication list yearly with the doctor) ... report problems."[22]

At every doctor's visit, take an up-to-date list of medications, including prescription, herbal, homeopathic, and over-the-counter drugs and vitamins. Some caregiving families may find it easier to put all Dad's medications in a sack and show it to the medical staff. Either method will inform his doctors of Dad's medicines.

Prescription Drugs with Increased Side Effects

Three types of medication have increased side effects: antibiotic (especially aminoglycosides), cancer and heart. "Many of these drugs have what doctors call a 'narrow therapeutic window.' In plain English, that means drugs for which the effective dose (the dose needed to treat your illness) is close to the toxic dose (the dose that can cause you harm)."[23]

Antibiotics, those miracle drugs which save lives, can cause problems if taken incorrectly. Over the decades since antibiotics were first developed, the American public began to expect their doctors to write a prescription for all infections. Meanwhile, the bacteria (germs) changed and mutated to survive all the antibiotics people were taking. As the germs became resistant, more potent antibiotics were needed and have been developed and a vicious cycle has occurred. Some bacteria have become "super" germs, able to survive many of the antibiotics available today. The result, as told by the American Academy of Family Physicians, is that "a few kinds of bacteria are resistant to all antibiotics and are now untreatable."[24]

The aminoglycoside family of medicines are a potent group of antibiotics which can cause harm to kidneys and can cause nerve damage resulting in deafness and blindness. These drugs are most commonly given intravenously and blood levels of the drug are monitored to prevent complications.

The American Academy of Family Physicians gives this information: "Antibiotics only work against infections caused by bacteria, fungi and certain parasites. They don't work against any infections caused by viruses. Viruses cause colds, the flu and most coughs and sore throat.... Do not expect antibiotics to cure every illness. Do not take antibiotics for viral illnesses, such as for colds or the flu. Often, the best thing you can do is let colds and the flu run their course. Sometimes this can take two weeks or more. If your illness gets worse after 2 weeks, talk to your doctor. He or she can also give you advice on what you can do to relieve symptoms while your body fights off the virus."[25]

Cancer medicines have a narrow therapeutic window because their purpose is to kill the cancer cells. A person undergoing cancer treatment, along with their caregivers, should ask for information about the drugs, desired action, and signs of toxicity or side effects. Cancer treatments often lower a person's immune system and make him more vulnerable to infection. Caregiving families should ask the doctor what signs and symptoms of infection they should watch for and report them to the doctor.

Heart and blood pressure medicines are the third type of medication which has serious side effects. Blood thinners such as heparin and warfarin (some with the brand name Coumadin) can cause bleeding and bruising. Heart arrthymic medicines such as digoxin can build up in a person's blood and cause the serious side effects of heart block, with a slow heart rate and low blood pressure. Some blood pressure/diuretic medicines can deplete the body of potassium and cause weakness and, if untreated, a life-threatening low potassium level. The caregiving family should learn about Mom and Dad's medicines, the desired action, the potential side effects and specific details associated with each medicine. Routine blood tests may be needed to monitor the blood levels of certain drugs.

Dad's doctor prescribed Coumadin to "thin" Dad's blood and prevent blood clots. Dad had atrial fibrillation, a heart rhythm problem which can cause blood clots. Dad began to get blood drawn at regular intervals to monitor the thickness of his blood. Dad's doctor would monitor the blood results and sometimes adjust the amount of Coumadin Dad was taking.

If Dad's blood level had gotten too thin, he would have been at risk for internal bleeding.

Caregiving families deal with medication issues for their loved ones. Resource people such as physicians and pharmacists provide valuable information to help these families cope.

Cost of Prescription Drugs

Prescription drugs can cost a lot of money, and the pharmaceutical companies are often criticized because of the expense of new drugs. However, it costs many millions of dollars to develop and bring a drug to the consumer.[26] Without the pharmaceutical companies and the medications they develop, the big three killers of 1900 might still be our major health problems.

Consumers can help control their prescription drug bills several ways. Ask the doctor and pharmacist if a generic version of the drug would be equal. What is a generic vs. a brand name drug? When new drugs are developed and brought to the consumer, they are marketed and advertised under the trade (brand) name the company chooses. For several years, this new drug is protected by patent and available only from that company and at the price the company charges. During these years, the company expects to earn back the money it spent on research and development of the drug. When the years of patent protection expires, other companies can then manufacture and sell the drug under different names, including a generic name. When the competition begins, pricing of the drug usually drops. Many generic drugs are comparable to the trade name versions. A doctor or pharmacist can give an opinion on the question of whether a generic version is available and would be as good. Generic drugs have another benefit: the side effects and benefits are well known because people have been using that drug for years. The U.S. Food and Drug Administration oversees development of both trade and generic drugs. People can rest assured that the generic drugs have been scrutinized by the FDA.

Generic drugs cost less. Many health insurance companies have tiered schedules of charges: brand name drugs have a higher co-pay (what the insured pays) and generic drugs have a smaller co-pay. Consumers can compare the prices of drugs at different pharmacies, as all pharmacies do not charge the same price. If a person wants to change pharmacies, he may need a new prescription written by his doctor to make that switch.

Buying in large quantities may save money. A person would need to check with his insurance plan and then have the doctor order the 90-day supply. Buying a 90-day supply instead of a 30-day supply might save money. Some medications can be supplied in a larger dose and divided. For example, a 20mg tablet which could be divided into two10 mg tablets might save money. This does not work for capsules or time-release medications which cannot be divided. Talk to a doctor about this option and purchase a tablet cutter from a pharmacy to ensure an evenly cut tablet and appropriate dosage from each tablet.

The medical world can be confusing to caregivers and their loved ones. A caregiver who better understands the medical world can better find the help he and his loved one needs.

Five Things You Can Do to Prevent Infection
(Courtesy the Joint Commission, non-profit U.S.-based organization responsible for accrediting health care programs)

1. Clean your hands.

Use soap and warm water. Rub your hands really well for at least 15 seconds. Rub your palms, fingernails, in between your fingers, and the backs of your hands.

Or, if your hands do not look dirty, clean them with alcohol-based hand sanitizers. Rub the sanitizer all over your hands, especially under your nails and between your fingers, until your hands are dry.

Clean your hands before touching or eating food. Clean them after you use the bathroom, take out the trash, change a diaper, visit someone who is ill, or play with a pet.

2. Make sure health care providers clean their hands or wear gloves.

Doctors, nurses, dentists and other health car providers come into contact with lots of bacteria and viruses. So before they treat you, ask them if they've cleaned their hands.

Health care providers should wear clean gloves when they perform tasks such as taking throat cultures, pulling teeth, taking blood, touching wounds or body fluids, and examining your mouth or private parts. Don't be afraid to ask them if they should wear gloves.

3. Cover your mouth and nose.

Many diseases are spread through sneezes and coughs. When you sneeze or cough, the germs can travel 3 feet or more. Cover your mouth and nose to prevent the spread of infection to others. Use a tissue! Keep tissues handy at home, at work and in your pocket. Be sure to throw away used tissues and clean your hands after coughing or sneezing.

If you don't have a tissue, cover your mouth and nose with the bend of your elbow or hands. If you use your hands, clean them right away.

4. If you are sick, avoid close contact with others.

If you are sick, stay away from other people or stay home. Don't shake hands or touch others.

When you go for medical treatment, call ahead and ask if there's anything you can do to avoid infecting people in the waiting room.

5. Get shots to avoid disease and fight the spread of infection.

Make sure that your vaccinations are current, even for adults. Check with your doctor about shots you may need. Vaccinations are available to prevent these diseases: chicken pox, measles, tetanus, shingles, flu (influenza), whooping cough (pertussis), German measles (rubella), pneumonia, human papillomavirus (HPV), mumps, diphtheria, hepatitis, and meningitis.

Know Your Rights: A Speak Up Initiative
(Courtesy the Joint Commission)

What are your rights?

You have the right to be informed about the care you will receive.

You have the right to get information about your care in your language.

You have the right to make decisions about your care, including refusing care.

You have the right to know the names of the caregivers who treat you.

You have the right to safe care.

You have the right to have your pain treated.

You have the right to know when something goes wrong with your care.

You have the right to get an up-to-date list of all of your current medicines.

You have the right to be listened to.

You have the right to be treated with courtesy and respect.

Ask for written information about all of your rights as a patient.

What is your role in your health care?
You should be active in your health care.
You should ask questions.
You should pay attention to the instructions given to you by your caregivers. Follow the instructions.
You should share as much information as possible about your health with your caregivers. For example, give them an up-to-date list of your medicines. And remind them about your allergies.

Can your family and friends help with your care?
Find out if there is a form you need to fill out to name your personal representative, also called an advocate. Ask about your state's laws regarding advocates.

How can an advocate help with your care?
They can get information and ask questions for you when you can't. They can remind you about instructions and help you make decisions. They can find out who to go to if you are not getting the care you need.

Can your advocate make decisions for you?
No, not unless they are your legal guardian or you have given them that responsibility by signing a legal document, such as a health care power of attorney.

Can other people find out about your disease or condition?
The law requires health care providers to keep information about your health private. You may need to sign a form if you want your health care providers to share information with your advocate or others.

What is "informed consent"?
This means that your health care providers have talked to you about your treatment and its risks. They have also talked to you about options to treatment and what can happen if you aren't treated.

What happens if something goes wrong during treatment or with my care?
If something goes wrong, you have the right to an honest explanation and an apology. The explanation and apology should be made in a reasonable amount of time.

How do you file a complaint?
First, call the hospital or health system so that they can correct the problem. Next, if you still have concerns, complaints can be sent to the

licensing authority or the Joint Commission, who provide a complaint form on their website at www.jointcommission.org.

Questions to ask before you enter the health care facility.
Can you have an advocate? Do you need to sign a document so your advocate can get important information about your care?
What can be done to make sure I don't get an infection?
Is there a form you need to sign about life-saving actions, like resuscitation?
Is there a form you need to sign about life support?
Does the organization allow members of your religion to visit and pray with you?
What kind of security does the facility have? Is there a 24-hour guard or alarm system?
Whom do you speak to if a problem arises? How does the organization handle complaints?
Are there any procedures that cannot be done at this facility for religious reasons?
Can you get a copy of your medical record and test results?

Tips for Your Doctor's Visit: Speak Up Initiative
(Courtesy the Joint Commission)

Talking with Your Doctor

What you can do to prepare for your doctor's visit.
Take all of your prescription and over-the-counter medicines, vitamins, and herbs with you when you visit the doctor. If you're unable to take them with you, take a current list of all the medicines, vitamins, and herbs that you take. Include how much you take.

Write down the following information to share with your doctor:
Your health history. Include allergies and bad reactions you have had to medicines, and the dates of any surgeries and hospital visits.
Your current health problems.
Any questions that you want to ask about your health.

What can you do if you don't understand what your doctor is saying?
Tell the doctor you do not understand. Ask more questions to help

the doctor understand what you need. Tell the doctor if you need someone who speaks your language or who knows sign language. Ask a trusted friend or family member to come with you.

What if you are too embarrassed to talk about your health problems?

It may help to write your health problems and symptoms down on paper to give to the doctor. A friend or family member may be able to help you talk to the doctor about your problem.

Ask about any new medicines your doctor prescribes.

Why do you need a new medicine? How will it help you?

What is the name of the medicine?

Is there a generic medicine you can take?

Is there a medicine on your insurance company's formulary that will work for you?

Is the medicine a liquid or a pill?

What are the directions for taking the medicine? Repeat the directions back to the doctor. Ask the doctor to write down the directions.

What are the side effects?

Can you take it with your current medicines? Should you stop taking any of your current medicines?

Should you avoid any foods or drinks when you take the medicine?

Would the medicine still work if you use half of it? As an example, can you cut a pill in half?

Remind your doctor about your allergies and reactions you have had to medicines. Tell the doctor if you don't understand any information about the medicine. Ask your doctor to give you an updated printed list of all medicines.

Why is the doctor asking personal questions?

The doctor needs to know about your habits so he or she can recommend the best treatment for you. Tell the doctor if you smoke, use recreational drugs, or are sexually active. The doctor can only talk to others about your health with your written permission.

Your doctor is sending you to another doctor — why?

Your doctor may send you to see a specialist. Specialists include heart doctors and doctors who treat cancer. Ask why the doctor recommends that you see another doctor.

Tips for the Examination

What can you do if you are uncomfortable being examined by the doctor?
Tell the doctor or nurse how you can be made more comfortable. Let them know if you would like a nurse or a family member or friend to stay with you.

Don't be afraid to ask the doctor or caregiver if they washed their hands.
Doctors, nurses and other caregivers usually wash their hands but they can forget. Remind them if you don't see them wash their hands. Hand washing helps prevent infection.

Make sure the doctor or caregiver wears clean gloves before examining you.
Ask them to wear clean gloves before giving shots, touching wounds, or examining your mouth or private parts.

If You Need a Lab Test

Questions to ask the doctor if you need a lab test:
Why is this test being done? What will it tell you about my health?
Are there any foods or drinks I should avoid before or after the test?
Should I take my medicine before the test?
Is there anything else I need to do to prepare for the test?
Are there any side effects of the test? Will it be painful or uncomfortable? Is it unusual to have pain or discomfort?
Should I have the test done before my next visit to the doctor?
Will I need someone to take me home after the test?

If You Need Treatment or Surgery

Find out about your condition and treatments for it.
Ask for written information about your conditions and treatments. Ask how and if a treatment will help you. Find out about risks of the treatments.

What can you do to prepare for your treatment?
Ask for copies of your health records from your doctor. Your records belong to you. It may take some time to get copies and there may be a cost.

Questions to ask the doctor if you need to have an operation:

Are there any vitamins, herbs, or prescription or over-the-counter medicines that you should not take before your operation?

Can you eat or drink before your operation?

Should you trim your nails and remove any nail polish?

After Your Doctor's Visit

Learn more about your condition.

Information can be found at the library, from support groups and reliable Web sites. Searching for a Web site is easy. Just type your disease or diagnosis into the search box on your computer's Internet search engine, such as Google.

What if you are not sure about the treatment or operation?

Make an appointment with another doctor to get a second opinion.

How can you find out if the hospital or facility you plan to go to is a good one?

Find out if the organization is accredited by the Joint Commission. Accredited means that the organization follows rules that guide safe and quality patient care. Visit the Joint Commission's Quality Check Web site at www.qualitycheck.org.

Talk to your doctor. Ask about the organization's experience taking care of people with your condition. How often do they perform the procedure you need? What special care do they provide to help patients get well.

Source: http://www.jointcommission.org/speak_up_tips_for_your_doctors_visit/.

Help Avoid Mistakes with Your Medicines: Speak Up Initiative
(Courtesy the Joint Commission)

Who is responsible for your medicines?

A lot of people — including you!

Doctors check all of your medicines to make sure they are OK to take together. They will also check your vitamins, herbs, diet supplements or natural remedies.

Pharmacists will check your new medicines to see if there are other medicines, foods or drinks you should not take with your new medicines. This helps to avoid a bad reaction.

Nurses and other caregivers may prepare medicines or give them to you.

You need to give your doctors, pharmacists and other caregivers a list of your medicines. This list should have your prescription medicines, over-the-counter medicines (for example, aspirin), vitamins, herbs, diet supplements, natural remedies, amount of alcohol you drink each day or week and recreational drugs.

What should you know about your medicines?

Make sure you can read the handwriting on the prescription. If you can't read it, the pharmacist may not be able to read it either. You can ask to have the prescription printed.

Read the label. Make sure it has your name on it and the right medicine name.

Make sure that you understand all of the instructions for your medicines.

If you have doubts about a medicine, ask your doctor, pharmacist or caregiver about it.

What if you forget the instructions for taking a medicine or are not sure about taking it?

Call your doctor or pharmacist. Don't be afraid to ask questions about any of your medicines.

What can you do at the hospital or clinic to help avoid mistakes with your medicines?

Make sure your doctors, nurses and other caregivers check your wristband and ask your name before giving you medicine. Some patients get a medicine that was supposed to go to another patient.

Don't be afraid to tell a caregiver if you think you are about to get the wrong medicine.

Know what time you should get a medicine. If you don't get it then, speak up.

Tell your caregiver if you don't feel well after taking a medicine. Ask for help immediately if you think you are having a side effect or reaction.

You may be given IV (intravenous fluids). Read the bag to find out what is in it. Ask the caregiver how long it should take for the liquid to run out. Tell the caregiver if it's dripping too fast or too slow.

Get a list of your medicines — including your new ones. Read the list carefully. Make sure it lists everything you are taking. If you're not well enough to do this, ask a friend or relative to help.

Questions to ask your doctor or pharmacist.
How will this new medicine help you?
Are there other names for this medicine? For example, does it have a brand or generic name?
Is there any written information about the medicine?
Can you take this medicine with your allergy? Remind your doctor about your allergies and reactions you have had to medicines.
Is it safe to take this medicine with your other medicines? Is it safe to take it with your vitamins, herbs and supplements?
Are there any side effects of the medicine? For example, upset stomach. Who can you call if you have side effects or a bad reaction? Can they be reached 24 hours a day, seven days a week?
Are there specific instructions for your medicines? For example, are there any foods or drinks you should avoid while taking it?
Can you stop taking the medicine as soon as you feel better? Or do you need to take it until it's gone?
Do you need to swallow or chew the medicine? Can you cut or crush it if you need to?
Is it safe to drink alcohol with the medicine?

Source: The Joint Commission, Help avoid mistakes with your medicines, http://www.jointcommission.org/speak_up_help_avoid_mistakes_with_your_medicines/pdf.

Personal Health Information Sheet

Name_____ Date_____
Primary Care Doctor_____ Date of last primary care doctor visit_____

Specialist I've seen/dates and reason
_____

Specialist I've seen/dates and reason
_____

Specialist I've seen/dates and reason
_____

Pharmacy I prefer to use & phone #
_____

Health insurance co._____Group #_____ Member #_____
Dental insurance co._____Group #_____ Member #_____
Vision insurance co._____Group #_____ Member #_____

Contact information in case of emergency (who should be called)
Name_____ Relationship_____
Address_____City & State_____
Home_____ Cell _____ Other phone _____

Secondary contact for emergency
Name_____ Relationship_____
Address_____City & State_____
Home_____ Cell _____ Other phone _____

Allergies to prescription medications/herbal medicines/latex/over-the-counter drugs
_____

Height_____ Weight_____ Blood Type_____

Current health conditions and symptoms (when symptoms started/description of symptoms/any treatments)
_____
_____

Current Medications (prescribed medications, herbal supplements, vitamins, over-the-counter drugs)

Medication name	Dosage & frequency	Date you started taking	Why you're taking med	What doctor prescribed it	Instructions (ex. Take before meals)

Past Medical History
Immunizations (Vaccinations)
Flu (influenza) shot_____ Hepatitis A_____
Hepatitis B_____ Measles/Mumps/Rubella_____
Chicken Pox_____ Pneumonia (Pneumococcal)_____
Tetanus, Diptheria_____ Meningitis (Meningococcus)_____
TB screen_____

Past Major Illness/Injury   Date   What happened   Treatment

_____
_____
_____

Past Hospitalizations   Date   Reason for   Treatment
                               hospital stay

_____
_____
_____

Surgery/Procedures   Date   Results

_____
_____
_____

Ongoing health problems	Doctor treating problem	When diagnosed	Past treatments	Treatments being done now

6. All Things Medical

Family Health History (Blood relatives)

How person was related to you	Major illnesses/ chronic ailments	Living or Deceased	If deceased, how old when relative died	What treatment was done	If deceased, what caused death

Health Examinations Done

Tests and exams	Date	What test or exam	Results
Eye exam/ Dental checkups			
Lab work such as cholesterol, blood chemistry levels, blood sugar levels, etc.			
Colon exams (occult blood screening, colonoscopy exam)			
Mammogram/ Bone Density test			
Dental exam			
Pelvic exam, Pap test (females)			
Testicular/Prostate exam (males)			

Recent lifestyle changes_____

Part I. Durable Power of Attorney for Health Care
(Courtesy Missouri Bar)

If you do *NOT* wish to name an agent to make health care decisions for you, write your initials in the box to the right and go to Part II.

Initials

This form has been prepared to comply with the "Durable Power of Attorney for Health Care Act" of Missouri.

1. **Selection of Agent.** I appoint:
   Name:_____
   Address:_____

   Telephone:_____
as my Agent.

2. **Alternate Agents.** Only an Agent named by me may act under this Durable Power of Attorney. If my Agent resigns or is not able or available to make health care decisions for me, of if an Agent named by me is divorced from me or is my spouse and legally separated from me, I appoint the person(s) named below (in the order named if more than one):

First Alternate Agent
Name:_____
Address:_____

Telephone:_____

Second Alternate Agent
Name: _____
Address:_____

Telephone:_____

THIS IS A DURABLE POWER OF ATTORNEY, AND THE AUTHORITY OF MY AGENT, WHEN EFFECTIVE, SHALL NOT TERMINATE OR BE VOID OR VOIDABLE IF I AM OR BECOME DISABLED OR INCAPACITATED OR IN THE EVEN OF LATER UNCERTAINTY AS TO WHETHER I AM DEAD OR ALIVE

6. All Things Medical

3. **Effective Date and Durability.** Except for such earlier dates as may be set forth in Section 4, below, this Durable Power of Attorney is effective when **two** physicians decide and certify that I am incapacitated and unable to make and communicate a health care decision.

- If you want ONE physician, instead of TWO, to decide whether you are incapacitated, write your initials in the box to the right.

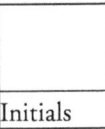

4. **Agent's Powers.** I grant to my Agent full authority to: |Initials|

A. Give consent to, prohibit or withdraw any type of health care, medical care, treatment or procedure, even if my death may result.

- If you wish to AUTHORIZE your Agent to direct a health care provider to withhold or withdraw artificially supplied nutrition and hydration (including tube feeding of food and water), write your initials in the box to the right. |Initials|

- If you DO NOT WISH TO AUTHORIZE your Agent to direct a health care provider to withhold or withdraw artificially supplied nutrition and hydration (including tube feeding of food and water), write your initials in the box to the right. |Initials|

B. Make all necessary arrangements for health care services on my behalf, and to hire and fire medical personnel responsible for my care;

C. Move me into or out of any health care facility (even if against medical advice) to obtain compliance with the decisions of my Agent; and

D. Take any other action necessary to do what I authorize here, including (but not limited to) any waiver or release from liability required by any health care provider, and taking any legal action at the expense of my estate to enforce this Durable Power of Attorney.

E. Act, effective immediately, as my "personal representative" as defined in 45 C.F.R. 164.502(g), the regulations enacted pursuant to the Health Insurance Portability and Accountability Act of 1996 ("HIPAA"), and as hereafter amended, for the purpose of authorizing the release of my complete health record as may be necessary in order to obtain for my benefit medical treatment or consultation.

5. Agent's Financial Liability and Compensation. My Agent acting under this Durable Power of Attorney will incur no personal financial liability. My Agent shall not be entitled to compensation for services performed under this Durable Power of Attorney, but my Agent shall be entitled to reimbursement for all reasonable expenses incurred as a result of carrying out any provision hereof.

Part II. Health Care Directive

If you DO NOT WISH to make a health care directive, write your Initials in the box on the right, and go to Part III.

[Initials]

I make this HEALTH CARE DIRECTIVE ("Directive") to exercise my right to determine the course of my health care and to provide clear and convincing proof of my wishes and instructions about my treatment.

If I am persistently unconscious and there is no reasonable expectation of my recovery from a seriously incapacitating or terminal illness or condition, I direct that all of the life-prolonging procedures that I have initialed below be withheld or withdrawn.

I want the following life-prolonging procedures to be withheld or withdrawn:

- **Artificially supplied nutrition and hydration (including tube feeding or food and water)**.......... _____ Initials

- **surgery or other invasive procedures**.................. _____ Initials

- **heart-lung resuscitation (CPR)**.......................... _____ Initials

- **antibiotic**... _____ Initials

- **dialysis**.. _____ Initials

- **chemotherapy**... _____ Initials

- **radiation therapy**.. _____ Initials

- **all other "life prolonging" medical or surgical procedures that are merely intended to keep me alive without reasonable hope of improving my condition or curing my illness or injury**................ _____ Initials

However, if my physician believes that any life-prolonging procedure may lead to significant recovery, I direct my physician to try the treatment for a reasonable period of time. If it does not improve my condition, I direct the treatment be withdrawn even if it shortens my life. I also direct that I be given medical treatment to relieve pain or to provide comfort, even if such treatment might shorten my life, suppress my appetite or my breathing, or be habit-forming.

I want to donate my organs or tissues and realize it may be necessary to maintain my body artificially after my death on a breathing machine until my organs can be removed.

Yes No I do not want to address this question now

IF I HAVE NOT DESIGNATED AN AGENT IN THE DURABLE POWER OF ATTORNEY, THIS DOCUMENT IS MEANT TO BE IN FULL FORCE AND EFFECT AS MY HEALTH CARE DIRECTIVE.

Part III. General Provisions Included in the Directive and Durable Power of Attorney

YOU MUST SIGN THIS DOCUMENT IN THE
PRESENCE OF TWO WITNESSES.

IN WITNESS WHEREOF, I have executed this document this ____day of _____(month), _____(year).

_____
Signature
Print Name _____
Address _____
_____

The person who signed this document is of sound mind and voluntarily signed this document in our presence. Each of the undersigned witnesses is at least eighteen years of age.

Signature_____ Signature_____
Print Name_____ Print Name_____
Address_____ Address_____
_____   _____

| ONLY REQUIRED FOR PART 1 — DURABLE POWER OF ATTORNEY |

STATE OF MISSOURI   )
)   SS
COUNTY OF _____   )

    On this _____ day of _____(month), _____(year), before me personally appeared _____, to me known to be the person described in and who executed the foregoing instrument and acknowledged that he/she executed the same as his/her free act and deed.

    IN WITNESS WHEREOF, I have hereunto set my hand and affixed my official seal in the County of _____, State of Missouri, the day and year first above written.

                                                                                   Notary Public

My Commission Expires:

7

All Things Surgical

Surgery Procedures — Emergency Surgery

Janet was walking her dog, Ginger, across her backyard when Janet tripped and fell. She found her leg would not work properly and she could not get up. Fortunately, she had her cell phone in her pocket so she called her daughter, who came to check on her. With her daughter's help, Janet was able to stand but felt pain when she put weight on her injured leg. A trip to the hospital emergency room was necessary. The workup in the ER found Janet's right hip was broken.

An orthopaedic surgeon came and talked to Janet. She was greatly relieved when she heard who was on call, a surgeon she had seen on prior occasions. As her surgeon talked to Janet and her family, he showed them her X-rays and explained what surgery would be right for her fracture. After this discussion, they all agreed with the surgeon's plan for Janet: she would have hip prosthesis surgery the next morning. Janet was transferred to the orthopaedic floor and settled in for the night. The next morning she had surgery to fix her broken right hip. The surgery and her recuperation went well.

After her surgery, Janet had to spend a few weeks at a rehabilitation facility recuperating while her main floor bathroom at home was remodeled. She learned how to use a walker because her doctor did not want her putting full weight on her hip or climbing stairs while it healed. She was happy when she returned home to recuperate and heal her broken hip.

An emergency occurs. When a person comes to a hospital emergency room, their actions (and maybe their words) are a request for help. They are hurting or injured and they expect medical personnel at the ER to do things to make them better and relieve the pain. The medical personnel get busy taking care of the person, drawing blood, hooking the person to monitors if needed, having X-rays taken in an effort to diagnose the problem, and taking appropriate steps to make the person better.

At the same time, family members are probably feeling stressed. They can feel overwhelmed as medical personnel start to take care of the injury or do tests to make a diagnosis. Blood is drawn and the person may be shuttled back and forth to the X-ray department for a variety of X-rays, CT scans or MRIs. The family may be allowed back with the person or, depending on the ER space, the family may have to stay in the waiting room. They sit there wondering what's going on with Mom as they check their watches for the hundredth time. The patient and family are feeling vulnerable. In this situation, they all find life spinning out of their control.

Preparing Before the Emergency Occurs

One way to decrease the stresses of emergencies is to prepare ahead of time. Most older people require surgery of some type at some time. Family and caregivers can be prepared. Everyone needs a primary care physician (family doctor). Chapter 6 gives suggestions on how to choose a doctor, surgeon(s) and a local hospital. Then when an emergency happens, it won't be stressful deciding which hospital to go to: "Mom always uses Hospital A, we will go there."

If Mom cannot fill out a personal health information sheet (see pages 98–101) then a family member can help fill it out. The first effort to fill out this information sheet will require the most effort and time. After that, keeping it current will be easier. Then if an emergency happens, family can grab a copy of that form and Mom's living will/advanced directive for health care for the hospital staff. A copy of those papers will be placed in Mom's chart for every hospital visit. The copy from the last hospitalization cannot be reused.

Caregivers may feel like they spend lots of time at the hospital with their elderly family members. Statistics agree. A 2006 National Hospital Discharge Survey compared hospitalization (inpatient) figures. In 1970, a total of 20 percent of hospital inpatients were older than 65 years. In 2006, 38 percent were over age 65.[1]

Elective Surgery

Elective surgery is a planned event. For example, a total knee replacement being performed for arthritis pain or cataract surgery would be considered elective, planned procedures. "In the mid–1900s, surgeons often hesitated to perform even simple operations on people over age 50. Times have changed! Now, more than one third of all operations in the United States are performed on people 65 and over."[2]

As surgery and anesthesia became safer, more of the over–65 group have surgery. Some of the most common elective surgical procedures for the over–65 group include cataract surgery and total joint replacements.

As elective surgery is a planned event, there's time to prepare beforehand. Wise caregivers will begin with asking what surgery Mom needs and educate themselves on the procedure. *Dr. David Scherer's HOSPITAL Survival Guide* gives the following suggestions: Ask the surgeon for brochures or information about the surgery he is proposing, read books on the topic, search reputable Internet sites, learn about nonsurgical alternatives (if available) to the proposed surgery and talk to other people who have had that procedure performed.[3]

Bill's arthritis was causing him so much pain that he stopped playing golf. After he sat around the house, bored out of his mind, for a month, his wife and daughter told Bill it was time to see his doctor. Bill saw his primary care doctor and was referred to an orthopaedic surgeon who could perform total joint surgery. When Bill saw the surgeon, the surgeon sat down and talked about Bill's knee X-ray and gave his recommendations for joint replacement surgery. He talked to Bill about the risks of complications and actions taken to decrease those risks. The surgeon gave him brochures from the Arthritis Foundation to read at home, ending with this: "I don't expect an answer today. You think about it and give us a call when you're ready to have surgery."

Bill's daughter got online at the Arthritis Foundation's "Surgery Center" to gather more information. Bill called a buddy who had undergone a total knee surgery a couple years before and asked his opinion. One afternoon Bill's wife went to their local library and borrowed a book on osteoarthritis that they read together. Bill's family learned about osteoarthritis and total knee replacement surgery. They were reassured to find the surgeon was recommending a procedure that matched the information they were reading.

Surgical Procedures — Laparoscopic, Minimally Invasive, Lasers and Robots

Words used to describe surgical procedures can be confusing. What do these mean to a caregiver?

Laparoscopy (also called keyhole surgery) has become a common procedure. Instead of a large abdominal incision (laparotomy) procedure, laparoscopy is done using scopes, cameras and long-handled, pencil-sized instruments. Several tiny incisions (approximately ½") are made in the abdominal wall. Carbon dioxide gas (the same gas humans exhale with every breath) is pumped into the abdomen to expand the abdominal wall during surgery and make it easier for the surgeon and staff to visualize and work safely with the specialized instruments. Laparoscopic procedures commonly performed include laparoscopic cholecystectomy (removal of the gallbladder), laparoscopic appendectomy (removal of the appendix) and laparoscopically assisted vaginal hysterectomy (removal of the uterus). The advantages of laparoscopy are the tiny incisions, less blood loss, quicker recovery (both discharge from the hospital and quicker return to normal activities) for the patient, and less pain because the large abdominal muscles aren't cut. Laparoscopic surgery patients often go home the day of surgery, or the next day in some cases, depending on the procedure performed and also the age and health of the patient.

The term "minimally invasive" is used for surgeries which have been modified to achieve smaller incisions and quicker recovery for the patient.

Lasers direct light beams to cut or destroy tissue and are used in many surgical procedures. A very popular eye surgery, LASIK, uses laser light beams to reshape the cornea, correcting eye conditions such as nearsightedness. Many people who formerly wore glasses enjoy no longer wearing them after a LASIK procedure. Lasers are usually a minimally invasive type of procedure.

The term "robot" brings to mind a short, round R2-D2 robot of *Star Wars* fame, but the robotic equipment used in surgery is different. The "robot" is a large machine with arms which straighten. The operating room scrub technician applies sterile drapes and attaches sterile surgical tools to these arms. Three-D telescopes, cameras and large video screens mounted on the operating room wall enable all staff within the room to see what the surgeon sees. The surgeon sits at a 3-D computer console and actively controls what the robotic equipment is doing. The robot "cannot make decisions, nor can it perform any type of movement or maneuver without the surgeon's direct input."[4] Procedures being done using the robotic equipment include prostatectomy (removal of part or all of the prostate), hysterectomy, and some open heart procedures, The advantages of robotic surgery is that it's a laparoscopic procedure with those advantages plus the quality of 3-D visualization (enlarged and crisp real-time visualization) and the ability of the robotic arm to move into positions a surgeon's wrist cannot.

These technological advances have made surgery less painful and the recovery time shorter, but these benefits carry an increased price tag because the initial cost of a robot is over $1 million plus annual upkeep.

Planning for Surgery

The person anticipating surgery, as well as his family will find the surgical process easier if a plan is made. Does Mom need her gallbladder removed? What procedure does the surgeon recommend? How long will recovery take and what limitations will she deal with? A family meeting, either in person or by e-mail and conference calls, can be used to get organized. A doctor's visit reveals this information: Mom will have a laparoscopic cholecystectomy and should be in the hospital 23 hours (that means she will stay in the hospital overnight and go home the next day). She will be limited to lifting a gallon of milk (nothing heavier) for a couple weeks after surgery. The surgeon reviewed Mom's medicine and told her to not take her gingko pills for a specific time before surgery to decrease the risk of postoperative bleeding.

When they heard this information, this family began to make plans. This family divided up the different aspects of care their mom would need. Her retired son who lived down the street volunteered to chauffeur Mom to all doctor appointments and to the hospital and to bring her home from the hospital; he would stay at the hospital the day of surgery and talk to the doctor after surgery. One of the daughters volunteered to stay with Mom the night of surgery in the hospital. Although the nurses were excellent, the family decided they wanted a family member to be with Mom the first night after surgery. This family also divided up the duties during Mom's recuperation period. They took turns bringing food to Mom's house when she got home. The grandson made sure her grass was mowed and her flowers were cared for during her recuperation. A teenage granddaughter (out of school for the summer) stayed at Mom's house several nights after she returned home; everyone felt better knowing someone would be in the house in case Mom needed help.

Preparing Home for Recuperation from Surgery

A person, and his family, contemplating surgery might need to prepare the home environment. Everyone needs a safe environment. Can throw rugs cause a fall? Is the house cluttered? A person considering total joint surgery might need to avoid stairs for a period of time. Can this person function on the main level without climbing steps? Does the main-level bathroom have a shower? Is the laundry room in the basement where the recuperating person cannot take care of laundry when she has recuperated and wants to resume doing her own laundry? A taller toilet or extension to the toilet would make using the toilet safer and easier. Does a home renovation need to be done to accommodate the recuperating person? More information about making the home environment safe for the elderly can be found in chapter 8.

Preparing One's Body for Surgery

The weeks prior to elective surgery can be used to make one's body healthy. Eat healthy meals and include lean proteins, complex carbohydrates, healthy fats, and vitamins, which are found in fruits and vegetables. The body will need these nutrients as it heals itself. Unless instructed by a surgeon to lose weight, preoperative and postoperative time frames are not the time to diet or starve. Better healing occurs when a person eats healthily and gives his body the building blocks needed to heal tissues.

Keep hydrated. Dehydration increases the risk of infection.[5] Most people should be drinking adequate amounts of water and noncaffeinated fluids in the days and weeks before surgery. Some people, such as kidney or congestive heart failure patients, will have fluid restrictions and should follow their doctor's recommendations.

Are teeth and gums healthy? Researchers have found there's a link between gingivitis and periodontal disease and inflammation, which can lead to arteriosclerosis and heart disease. More details on this topic can be found in chapter 10, "Aging Gracefully."

Many doctors believe that gingivitis/periodontal disease raises the risk of infection for any implanted medical device. Any person anticipating a surgery with implants, such as total joint replacement, should talk to the surgeon before surgery. Good questions to ask the surgeon would be these: "Should I have my dental examination and teeth cleaning before surgery?

How long before surgery should this be performed? Should I have antibiotics for future teeth cleaning after total joint surgery?"

Are there signs of infection on a person's body? Is that ingrown toenail red, swollen and painful? Did that itchy mosquito bite turn into a swollen, reddened, tender sore? Intact, healthy skin is considered an important defense against infection. A person who develops signs of infection (a reddened, swollen, painful sore or a weeping open sore) needs to notify the surgeon before any surgery is performed. Any white/yellow or green discharge from a sore should be discussed with the surgeon and appropriately treated. If a person develops a fever and begins to feel "sick," feeling bad, tired or exhausted, he needs to notify the surgeon of it before surgery is performed. Any acute respiratory infection with symptoms such as runny nose, sore throat, and cough should be discussed with the surgeon. The surgeon will decide whether to proceed with surgery as scheduled or postpone it until the patient has recovered from the respiratory infection.

Researchers believe that depression weakens the immune system. Often people who are depressed also indulge in unhealthy behaviors such as increased smoking, drinking alcohol, drinking caffeine, making unhealthy food choices, sleeping poorly and avoiding physical exercise.[6] The person who is feeling down and depressed should discuss this situation with his doctor or surgeon before undergoing surgery.

People who deal with diabetes and high blood sugar issues should recognize that high blood sugars contribute to postoperative infections. In a September 2010 *Archives of Surgery* article, researchers call a person's high blood sugar "the most important risk factor for SSI (surgical site infections)." Caregivers should work with their doctor (or their loved one's doctor) to control blood sugar levels and help prevent postoperative infections.[7]

Anesthesia Issues

The advancement of safety and pain control through the specialty of anesthesia can be found in chapter 5 of this book. Because of past and continuing improvements, people readily accept the risks of undergoing anesthesia for surgery.

Who gives anesthesia? Anesthesiologists and certified registered nurse anesthetists (CRNAs). Anesthesiologists are specialty doctors who spend extra years becoming experts on anesthesia and pain control. CRNAs are registered nurses who have extra schooling (a master's degree) and training to become proficient at anesthesia and pain control.

The preoperative interview with an anesthesiologist or CRNA looks at the whole person. The anesthesiologist will look at the function of a person's vital organs such as the heart, lungs, kidneys and brain.

Mr. H had a recent heart attack and he faces increased risks. An anesthesiologist would weigh those risks and choose the safest, most effective anesthesia for him. The anesthesiologist reviewing Mr. H's lab work, EKG and chest X-rays would consider all the possible problems which could happen during Mr. H's surgery and make recommendations. He might say, "I see you're having a total knee surgery. Since you had a heart attack a few months ago, the safest anesthesia for you will be a regional block. I would recommend a spinal anesthesia. What do you think about that plan?"

The three major types of anesthesia are general anesthesia, regional anesthesia and local anesthesia. When an anesthesiologist, a CRNA or both administer anesthesia to a patient, they will continuously monitor vital signs, give medications and appropriate anesthesia treatments to provide safe anesthesia care to that patient through the surgery and postoperative phase of a person's recovery.

General anesthesia involves the person becoming unconscious and unaware during the surgery. The anesthesia drugs are given through an intravenous (IV) line in a person's vein and the gases or vapors are inhaled through a breathing mask attached to the anesthesia machine.

Regional anesthesia includes spinal and epidural blocks. The anesthesia care provider injects the medications for these blocks into an area of the body (usually the back) and numbs the nerves which affect the surgical site. Many expectant mothers want epidural blocks during the birth of a child. It decreases or eliminates the pain of giving birth while allowing the awake mother to participate in the birth of her child. During regional anesthesia, a person can be sedated and nap through the procedure or the person can be awake.

Local anesthesia is used for minor procedures because the numbing medicine is injected directly into the tissue being operated upon. Local anesthesia works fine for superficial procedures. The person receiving local anesthesia would be awake unless some sedation was given to enable him to nap through the procedure.

Prevent Infections While in the Hospital and at Home

"Skin and mucous membranes are highly effective physical barriers against microorganisms."[8] Mucous membranes are the lining surface of the gastrointestinal, respiratory and genitourinary canals. For example, the tissue lining visible inside the mouth is mucous membrane. Healthy skin and mucous membranes protect against germs, viruses and other harmful microscopic organisms. People undergoing surgery usually have incisions made in their skin. Beginning a surgical experience with healthy intact skin increases the probability that infection-free recovery will follow.

How do the surgeons and operating room staff prevent infections in their patients? During time in the operating room, the surgeon and operating room staff follow aseptic (absence of sepsis or germs) technique. This means instruments are sterile. The patient's skin is scrubbed or painted with antiseptic solutions known to kill germs and viruses. Many evidence-based behaviors practiced by the surgeon and surgical staff contribute to an infection-free result for their patients.

The Joint Commission gives this advice about five things you can do to prevent infection: wash/clean your hands ... make sure health care providers wash/clean their hands or wear gloves ... cover your mouth and nose for a cough or sneeze ... if you are sick, avoid being close to others ... get vaccination shots to avoid disease and fight the spread of infection.[9]

Hand washing continues to be an easy, inexpensive weapon in the fight to prevent infections. Everyone, including family members, involved with a surgical patient should practice proper hand washing to protect the patient. According to the Centers for Disease Control, the following is the correct way to wash one's hands: hold hands under clean running (if possible warm) water, apply soap, rub hands together to lather all surfaces for 15 to 20 seconds (sing "Happy Birthday" twice to approximate the 20-second time frame); rinse hands under running water and dry hands with a paper towel or air dryer; use a paper towel to turn off the faucet and open the bathroom door as you leave the bathroom.

When one's hands aren't visibly soiled, an alcohol-based hand rub can be used to kill germs and prevent infections. The proper way to use alcohol-based hand sanitizer is to apply the product to the palm of one's hand and rub the hands together, covering all surfaces until the hands are dry.[10]

People are sent home quickly after surgery, often the same day. Frequently the instructions received at the hospital say to keep the dressing clean and dry until the patient sees the doctor at the first office visit. That means leave the dressing in place, dry and intact. One woman draped her operative hand with dressing on the top of the shower door to keep it away from water. Her husband had to help her but she accomplished a shower and kept the dressing on her hand dry. If the nursing staff at the hospital gives other instructions, the caregiver should begin with hand washing, then follow the instructions for wound care that the nursing staff gave them. Afterwards, the caregiver should dispose of old dressings in the trash and wash his hands thoroughly.

Preadmission Testing and Teaching (PATT)

The final part of planning for elective surgery involves the preoperative testing and teaching, which takes place at the hospital, medical center, or clinic. People who are scheduled for surgery must go for PATT before surgery. The preoperative testing is ordered by the surgeon and anesthesiologist and will vary. A young healthy person's surgeon may not order any blood tests or X-rays. Patients with more complicated health histories and chronic diseases may need several blood tests and X-rays.

If ordered by the surgeon, some of the common blood work tests done include a complete blood count (CBC), chem-7 (lists 7 indicators of a person's health status), clotting times, and a urine analysis. A CBC shows white blood cells (WBC), red blood cells (RBC), and platelets.

When elevated, white blood cells (leukocytes) can indicate infection, inflammatory processes, severe tissue damage, or leukemia. A low white blood cell count can indicate an autoimmune process, bone marrow failure or liver or spleen disease. There are multiple types of WBCs and they function in different ways. Some WBCs fight infectious invaders of the body. Others respond during an allergic reaction. A normal WBC count is 4,800 to 10,800 cells/mcL.

Red blood cells (erythrocytes) carry hemoglobin, the oxygen carrier of the body. A higher than normal number of RBCs can indicate conditions which include dehydration, kidney disease, and smoking. A low number of RBCs indicates anemia from a variety of causes, including hemorrhage, kidney failure, bone marrow failure, malnutrition, and autoimmune diseases. Hematocrit indicates the percentage of the blood composed of RBCs. The RBC count varies between males and females and may vary with altitude:

> Normal RBC count for males: 4.2 to 5.4 million cells/mcL
> Normal Hematocrit count for males: 40 to 50 percent
> Normal Hemoglobin for males: 14 to 16.5 gm/dL
> Normal RBC count for females: 3.6 to 5.0 million cells/mcL
> Normal Hematocrit count for females: 37 to 47 percent
> Normal Hemoglobin for females: 12.0 to 15.0 gm/dL

Platelets (thrombocytes) are necessary for blood clotting. Without platelets and the body's ability to form blood clots, even a small injury would result in hemorrhage. A low number of platelets can indicate chemotherapy, conditions such as hemolytic anemia, disseminated intravascular coagulation (DIC) or leukemia. An elevated number of platelets may indicate conditions such as anemia or certain types of cancer. A normal platelet count is 150,000 to 400,000/mcL.[11]

A patient's surgeon or anesthesiologist may order an ECG for people over age 40 or people with a history of heart problems. An EKG gives a tracing which shows the electrical activity of the heart. If a person has had a recent heart attack with damage, an EKG abnormality should show up. An EKG is a noninvasive procedure which is painless and takes five minutes to accomplish. A technician applies sticky leads to multiple places over the person's body and turns on the machine, which records the electrical activity of the heart.

A chest X-ray may be ordered to verify the health of a person's chest, including his heart and lungs. This X-ray gives a black-and-white image of the chest and the structures within it. A doctor could diagnose a person's pneumonia by looking at that person's chest X-ray. Rib fractures or bony abnormalities of the chest would show up on a chest X-ray.

Chem-7 is another blood test a doctor might order. The blood for this test would be drawn when that for a CBC is drawn. The chem-7 metabolic panel measures blood sugar (glucose), electrolyte and fluid balance and kidney function. Normal results of a chem-7 test follow:

Sodium	135–145 mEq/L
Potassium	3.5–5.0 mEq/L
Chloride	98–106 mmol/L
Carbon dioxide	20–29 mmol/L
Glucose	less than 100 mg/dL
Blood urea nitrogen (BUN)	8–20 mg/dL
Creatinine	0.6–1.2 mg/dL[12]

Clotting time tests will be performed if a person routinely takes a "blood thinner." Before a person undergoes surgery, the surgeon may want a clotting test done to verify the blood thinner is out of the patient's system and that normal blood clotting will occur. A normal prothrombin time (protime or PT) results are 11 to 13.5 seconds.[13] INR indicates the active nature of the blood thinner and is included with the PT test. An INR for a healthy person not on blood thinner is 1.0 or less. When a person is on anticoagulants, the INR number is larger, up to 4.0 for some medical conditions.[14] Normal partial thromboplastic (PTT) time is 25 to 35 seconds.[15]

A urine test shows basic kidney function and also shows if a kidney infection is present. This test may be ordered for some surgical patients.

The anesthesiologist will see the patient during this PATT visit. After reviewing the surgery planned and the patient's health history, the anesthesiologist will discuss the recommended plan for surgery and might say, "After reviewing your record, I recommend general anesthesia for your planned surgery. You should take your usual morning medicines with a sip of water. Other than that, you should stop eating at 8 P.M. the night before and stop drinking at midnight." The anesthesiologist would discuss the risks of anesthesia and ask the patient if he approves of the anesthesia plan.

The preoperative teaching involves instructions for preparing for surgery. The PATT nurses may provide written instructions and review those instructions with the patient and family. The nurse might say, "Leave all jewelry and valuables at home. You can eat till 8 P.M. the night before surgery and drink till midnight. After those times, please do not eat or drink except to take your morning medicines with a sip of water. Take a shower the night before with this special soap we're sending with you. Please be here at 6 A.M.; let them know at the Registration Center when you arrive."

The Day of Surgery

The day of surgery can be one long day. In an effort to minimize the waiting, patients are often given a time to be at the facility. The first patients arriving in the morning will be the first patients to have surgery that day. The patients scheduled for later in the day will be given later times to arrive. Even so, the day of surgery can still be a long one.

"The patient should expect to give his name and birthday to staff members repeatedly at the hospital. This identification may feel cumbersome at times, but the purpose is patient safety."[16] As a part of the registration process, a name band will be placed on the patient's arm. The patient will be given a hospital gown and asked to remove his clothes, his belongings to be cared for by family or hospital staff. The patient will be asked to lie on a cart and warm blankets will be provided. As a part of this process, the patient will be asked to sign permits for the surgery, administration of anesthesia and blood transfusions if they are needed.

After the patient is comfortable, the nurse will check and record vital signs, including blood pressure, heart rate, temperature and respirations. A pulse oxymetry finger clip will be placed on one of the patient's fingers. This monitor tells that the patient is breathing enough to keep his blood oxygenated. After all preliminary work is finished, the patient receives preoperative medications ordered by the anesthesiologist during the PATT interview. Routines vary in different hospitals, but routine preoperative medications may include an anti-ulcer medication such as famotide (Pepcid) and a relaxing medicine such as midazolam hydrochloride (Versed) and an antinausea drug such as dolasetron (Anzemet). All these medications go into the IV line that the nurse inserts into a vein, usually in the hand or forearm.

If the surgery site involves laterality (a left leg or right arm) or a specific level of the spine for back surgery, the surgeon will place his mark on the operative site before the patient is taken to the operating room. Some surgeons routinely greet their patient in the holding room before the patient is taken to the OR.

At any time if the patient is chilly, he should speak up and ask for warm blankets. Being warm is more comfortable and contributes to an infection-free operation.

The patient may not remember going to the operating room because of the medication he has received. In the operating room, the patient is moved over to the bed and monitors are attached. Routine monitoring done in the operating room includes EKG, pulse oxymetry and blood pressure. The anesthesia care provider will begin giving the anesthesia and might say, "Pick out a nice dream. You're going to sleep and we will be with you all the time."

After Surgery

The next thing the patient will know is waking up in the post anesthesia care unit (PACU) or "recovery room." The patient will be closely monitored during the stay in the PACU, approximately an hour. The nursing staff will stay close, monitor vital signs and talk with the patient often. If the patient feels pain, nausea, chilly or any other discomforts, he should speak up so the nurses can fix the problems. Pain control is important, and the nurses will ask if the patient is hurting and to rate the pain. The PACU nurses can give pain medication when their patients need it.

When the patient is awake and vital signs are stable, he will be moved to the nursing floor if he's staying overnight or to the step-down recovery room if he's going home. Family members are allowed to visit now. If the patient is going to the nursing floor for overnight, the patient is settled in there comfortably. Nurses will check on him frequently, monitoring vital signs and watching over his continued recovery. If the patient is going home, the nurses continue monitoring vital signs and making the patient comfortable but the goal is to return home that day.

Postoperative Teaching and Instructions

Before being released from the hospital, the patient and family are given instructions such as how to care for the surgical incision and how to control any pain the patient experiences. These instructions are important to prevent complications. If the patient or family has any questions, they should ask them at this time. A copy of the postoperative instructions should be sent home with the patient and family and should include phone numbers and a contact person who can answer any questions which arise after the patient gets home.

Returning home after elective surgery should be fairly straightforward because the family has had time to plan this event. They've divided the chores and they simply put their plan into action. The family dealing with a return home after emergency surgery may find themselves scrambling. Issues to be considered involve the physical layout of the home. Can Mom get into and out of the house easily or must she navigate steps? Must she climb steps to get to the bedroom? If so, can a temporary bedroom be set up downstairs? Does Mom live alone? Who can stay with her while she recuperates? Who can provide food for her? Who can drive her to her doctors' appointments and therapy appointments?

These questions can overwhelm the caregiving family. A family conference (in person or by phone) would benefit this family as they begin to make a plan to care for Mom during her recuperation. The primary caregiver might offer suggestions of what would be most helpful that out-of-town members can contribute to her care. Friends who make offers to help can be welcomed with suggestions like, "I know you love to garden. Do you think you could come by a couple times over the next month and care for Mom's flowers? She would appreciate the help and enjoy a visit from you also."

Some people may need various therapies which could delay their going home. A person whose split-level home makes getting around difficult might find a short stay at the rehabilitation wing of a hospital or nursing home beneficial. Therapies such as occupational therapy would teach him to walk with a walker or cane. Physical therapy would strengthen his body to help him with balance and prevent falls when he returns home. Social workers and discharge planner nurses at the hospital will assist the patient and family in making arrangements for needed therapies. The person who is going home might find that home health nursing staff is needed. This service would also be ordered by the surgeon and arranged by social workers/discharge planners at the hospital.

Recuperation takes time. The patient and family should realize that healing takes time. Even a person who had a laparoscopic surgery needs time to heal and recuperate. Even that person may hear his surgeon impose limitations. For example, the surgeon might say, "No lifting anything over a gallon of milk" for a certain period of time. Good advice for the postoperative healing phase involves being patient with oneself, eating a healthy diet and preventing infections. After surgery, a person may feel tired and listless. One who has undergone surgery should expect to have good days and bad days, which over time should improve to more good days and fewer bad days.

Eating a healthy diet gives the body nutrients it needs to heal and regain strength. Some people may experience a poor appetite. If a lack of appetite persists, the patient and family should consult the patient's doctor about this problem. The surgeon may recommend a milkshake type dietary supplement to provide the nutrition needed for healing.

Prevent infections in the surgical incision. Follow the surgeon's instructions. The surgeon may say to keep the dressing dry and do not remove it as his staff will change the dressing at the office visit. Or the surgeon may give instructions on how to change the dressing daily. Anyone who cares for the surgical wound, changes or handles the dressings should wash his hands before and after handling the dressings. "Hand washing is recommended by the Centers for Disease Control (CDC) as the best prevention of infections."[17] The surgeon wants to be notified of any signs and symptoms of infection: increasing redness, tenderness or swelling of the incision, any drainage from the incision, or chills and fever above 100.5 degrees Fahrenheit.

A wise patient and family will follow the instructions their surgeon gives them, and they will get the best results when they do so.

Help Avoid Mistakes in Your Surgery: Speak UP Initiative

(Courtesy the Joint Commission, non-profit U.S.-based organization responsible for accrediting health care programs)

Preparing for Your Surgery

Ask your doctor

Are there any prescription or over-the-counter medicines that you should not take before your surgery?

Can you eat or drink before your surgery?

Should you trim your nails and remove any nail polish?

If you have other questions, write them down. Take your list of questions with you when you see your doctor.

Ask someone you trust to

Take you to and from the surgery facility.

Be with you at the hospital or surgery facility. This person can make sure you get the care you need to feel comfortable and safe.

Before you leave home:

Shower and wash your hair. Do not wear makeup. Your caregivers need to see your skin to check your blood circulation.

Leave your jewelry, money and other valuables at home.

At the Surgery Facility

The staff will ask you to sign an informed consent form. It lists:
- Your name
- the kind of surgery you will have
- the risks of your surgery
- that you talked to your doctor about the surgery and asked questions
- and that you agree to have the surgery.

Make sure everything on the form is correct. Make sure all of your questions have been answered. If you do not understand something on the form — speak up.

For your safety, the staff may ask you the same question many times. They will ask:
- Who you are
- What kind of surgery you are having

The part of your body to be operated on
They will also double-check the records from your doctor's office.

Before your surgery

A health care professional will mark the spot on your body to be operated on. Make sure they mark only the correct part and nowhere else. This helps avoid mistakes.

Marking usually happens when you are awake. Sometimes you cannot be awake for the marking. If this happens, a family member or friend or another health care worker can watch the marking. They can make sure that your correct body part is marked.

Your neck, upper back or lower back will be marked if you are having spine surgery. The surgeon will check the exact place on your spine in the operating room after you are asleep.

Ask your surgeon if they will take a "time out" just before your surgery. This is done to make sure they are doing the right surgery on the right body part on the right person.

After your surgery

Tell your doctor or nurse about your pain. Hospitals and other surgical facilities that are accredited by the Joint Commission must help relieve your pain.

Ask questions about medicines that are given to you, especially new medicines. What is it? What is it for? Are there any side effects? Tell your caregivers about any allergies you have to medicines. If you have more questions about a medicine, talk to your doctor or nurse before taking it.

Find out about any IV (intravenous) fluids that you are given. These are liquids that drip from a bag into your vein. Ask how long the liquid should take to "run out." Tell the nurse if it seems to be dripping too fast or too slow.

Ask your doctor if you will need therapy or medicines after you leave the hospital. Ask when you can resume activities like work, exercise and travel. Source: The Joint Commission, Speak Up: Help Avoid Mistakes in Your Surgery, http://www.jointcommission.org/speak_up_help_avoid_mistakes_in_your_surgery/.

Tell Your Doctor About ALL Supplements Before Surgery

Common Herbal Supplements	Uses	Possible Problems from HerbalDrugs During Surgery
Chamomile	Decrease gas & indigestion Relieve insomnia	Bleeding
Echinacea	Treat infections	Bleeding, cause allergic reaction, decreases effects of steroids
Ephedra (Ma huang)	Asthma Increase energy Decrease appetite	High blood pressure, insomnia, irregular heart rates/beats, stroke Heart attack/death, seizures
Feverfew	Headaches Fever Psoriasis	Bleeding (decreased platelet function) overreact with vasoactive anesthesia drugs
Garlic	Treat cholesterol Lower blood pressure Antibacterial Bronchitis	Bleeding
Ginger	Nausea, indigestion, motion sickness	Bleeding
Gingko	Poor memory, diabetes, poor circulation	Bleeding Increased intracranial pressure
Ginseng	Anti-stress, fatigue, viral infections	Bleeding, low blood sugar, high blood pressure, prolong blood thinner warfarin

Kava	Anxiety, sedative	Strengthens anesthetic drugs, barbiturates/narcotics
Licorice	Arthritis, asthma, poor appetite, stomach ulcers, cough suppressant	High blood pressure Retain salt & water/edema
St. John's wort	Depression, anxiety	Prolong anesthesia drugs Increase drug metabolism
Valerian	Nerves, depression, insomnia	Strenthen anesthesia & central nervous system drugs & narcotics
Vohimbe	Impotence	Decrease anesthesia effects, cause tremors, fast heart rate/high blood pressure

Sources: MacKichan, C., and J. Ruthman (2004). "Herbal product use and perioperative patients." AORN Journal 79(5), 948–959.

DeLamar, L.M. (2005). "Preparing Your Patient for Surgery." *Topics in Advanced Practice Nursing eJournal* 5(1). http://www.medscape.com/viewarticle/500887_print (accessed 03/29/2005).

8

Practical Decisions

Dad Joseph has been in the hospital for almost two weeks with pneumonia. A family member has stayed with Mom Kathryn day and night. One sibling who lives several hours away just returned to his home after a week of being with Kathryn. Both sisters who live close by have run themselves ragged trying to work and wait on the folks. Nerves are stretched and tempers are short. Out-of-town sibling calls his sibling "Sister Sergeant" because she has taken charge. When in-charge daughter tells Kathryn to get ready for her beauty shop appointment in 10 minutes, Kathryn responds smartly. Daughter ends up in tears, or as she calls it "a meltdown." Almost two weeks of stress and strain has worn everyone down. The elderly parents are worried about each other and want to be at home together. The adult children are caring for both parents, juggling visitation times, meetings with doctors and therapists and their job responsibilities.

The timing was the holiday season. Joseph became ill before Thanksgiving. His illness encompassed Christmas, New Year's and most of January. That year's holiday season found the adult children and their families spending every available moment at the hospital. Everyone rode the roller coaster of hope and despair as Joseph struggled to recover from pneumonia.

In week four of being in the hospital (a few days after Christmas), Joseph moved to a rehabilitation hospital. He recognizes how close he came to dying and tells everyone he's so grateful to God for sparing his life. However, now he faces the tough part of getting well enough to go home. His lungs aren't healthy and he needs high levels of oxygen constantly to be comfortable. The doctors are telling him and his family that he cannot go home needing oxygen at a level of 10–15 liters/minute. The pulmonary specialist and respiratory therapists work to assist Joseph in his recovery. Physical therapists walk him twice a day. He makes slow but steady progress for a few days, then his progress stops.

His motivation to get home with Kathryn wanes as he realizes he cannot force his body to get well. The adult children watch and worry, supporting and cheering every step of the way. Kathryn moves into one daughter's home and flourishes, enjoying the love and support of her family. But she's worried about Joseph. She wonders if she can take care of Joseph when he gets home. As Kathryn's health became more frail the last few years, Joseph had picked up the slack and had done more chores around the house. He was the family driver and he did the grocery shopping.

At week six, Joseph's future looks bleak. His fever has returned and his cough has gotten worse. His family had made arrangements for him to go home with hospice care. His discharge is postponed again because he is weak and sick. In spite of three rounds of antibiotics, Joseph can't seem to overcome the pneumonia.

In the last two weeks, Joseph has recognized he can't get well. He asks for his lawyer to update his and Kathryn's will and put his legal and financial affairs in order. Joseph weeps as he tells his children good-bye and asks them to "take care of your mother." Two days later, Joseph dies peacefully in his sleep.

Joseph's family says, looking back at this time, that they found having to deal with legal and financial matters increased their stresses. Joseph's family lawyer told them he would visit Joseph at the rehab hospital. The lawyer continued, "There are only two people I would make this effort to help and your dad is one of them."

This family recommends that elderly parents get their legal and financial affairs in order before a crisis happens. They found themselves dealing with their father's illness during the busy holiday season and the need for updating the legal and financial situation increased their stresses and cares.

The American Bar Association book, *You and Your Aging Parents*, gives help and insight into dealing with legal matters. The laws vary in different states and countries. A consultation with an elder-law attorney where the elder parent resides can direct families correctly. Do they need a will or a trust? Do they need a power of attorney for property and financial matters? This is a different document from a durable power of attorney for healthcare. Who will be the power of attorney for property?

A power of attorney "is a document that allows one person, the principal, to designate another person, the agent (or attorney in fact), to obtain private information and make decisions on the principal's behalf. For instance, you might give your accountant or lawyer power of attorney to obtain documents and take certain actions on your behalf."[1] During a hospitalization, the elder parent's POA could pay bills and do banking for him until the parent recovers and can take care of his own business affairs. When an elder parent can no longer care for his business affairs, the person with power of attorney can take care of the business for him.

You and Your Aging Parents gives valuable information about legal, financial and health care issues. Whether it's a will or a trust, a guardianship or a conservatorship, the book gives easy-to-understand information and reputable resources for managing this complex, important part of caregiving.

Finding Resources

How does a caregiving family find resources and where do they start? Jessica Hill works with the 211 network and she shares the following information about it: A call to the 211 network is free and confidential. Anyone can call for their own benefit or on behalf of someone else. In fact, they often hear from case managers, teachers and members of the clergy calling on behalf of others who aren't able to call for themselves.

The largest number of 211 calls involves a need for finances for basic needs such as food, rent money and utilities. The 211 specialists also help people find low-cost legal care, child care, adult day care, domestic violence help and even job-finding services. The 211 specialists are trained as crisis-line counselors. Sometimes people are in a situation and feeling overwhelmed; they can't tell you exactly what they need. The 211 specialist can listen as the person talks through his issue and can identify points where assistance is available.

When someone calls for help, he will hear a recording say to have pen and paper ready. The person needs to be ready to write because the 211 specialist is going to give a lot of information. Typically the 211 specialist tries to give three referrals, one of which is probably the best. They like for a person to have options. These highly trained specialists provide access to available resources. They give each agency's eligibility requirements and what fees may be charged. Many of the programs are free or have a sliding scale cost based on financial circumstances, but they let you know what the fees are, if any. The specialist will tell you the hours of operation for the agency — information a person needs to feel prepared to make that call to an agency and ask for their service.

If a caller doesn't feel he can make another phone call or manage an automated phone system, he should ask for help. The 211 specialist can make a 3-way call, navigating the system until he connects with an individual at the resource agency and say, "I'm from 211 and I have someone on the line for you" before transferring the call.

Another way to access the 211 network is online at www.211.org. The Website access asks for a person's zip code and/or city so local resources can be accessed. On the website the person can find toll free phone numbers to call. A caregiving family member who lives in Ohio can learn what resources are available where Mom lives in Minneapolis, MN, and what number to call for resources in that area.

The 211 network is a grassroots program; there's no national office with affiliate sites. Usually a local United Way or other service agency within a community starts a 211 program. They get permission from their state to be designated as a 211 site, which are accredited nationally by the Alliance of Information and Referral Systems through standards in place for how a 211 must operate.

Sometimes a caregiver and family may want reassurance that they're doing all they can to provide care. They may want to call 211 and say, "We're utilizing this agency. Is there anything that would help us? Is there anything else we should know about?" The 211 network can provide information to a caregiver who could benefit from a support group. Many caregivers find practical help, good advice and comfort in knowing other people are dealing with caregiving issues.

Jessica ends the interview by saying that, "211 is definitely the best starting place. The Area Agency on Aging offices provide a 'help line' but if a person's caregiving needs involve a child, the agency of aging probably won't be the place to get help. Two-one-one may refer a family to another agency, but it's a great place to start. Every 211 website usually gives alternate phone numbers including toll-free number. Also 211 is available 24/7. A family can call on Christmas Day and their call will be answered."[2]

Another good resource is the local Area Agency on Aging office. Anyone with internet access can locate phone numbers for it at http://www.eldercare.gov/ by "Search by Location." Another way to access Area Agency on Aging resources is through their toll free help line at 1-800-392-8771. Area Agency on Aging offices may offer a variety of services. In fact, each Area Agency on Aging office tailors its services to the needs of its area's residents. The needs of a large city population might be totally different from what people need who live in a rural area of the country.

Practical Decisions — Can Dad Continue to Live at Home?

How can caregivers assist the loved one who wants to continue living at home? They must recognize it's wise to organize family and friends into a group who will help Dad continue to do so. In some situations, these people will enable Dad to live at home by taking care of his yard work. In other situations, Dad needs someone to clean his house and cook his meals. What does Dad need? A needs assessment can give insight into how to best help Dad. A variety of professionals, including social workers and geriatric care managers, can help with a needs assessment. Family members can begin by considering the activities of daily living.

Activities of Daily Living

Can Dad feed himself? Can he dress and undress himself? Six mobility and personal care tasks, called "activities of daily living," involve feeding, dressing, bathing, toileting, walking and moving from a bed to a chair. These six tasks are necessary parts of independent living. A person who cannot accomplish these tasks cannot function independently.

Instrumental Activities of Daily Living

The instrumental activities of daily living involve tasks such as using the telephone, grocery shopping, preparing meals, housework, laundry, taking medications, managing money, and transportation issues. The IADL tasks are chores that family and friends can perform.[3]

Raymond wanted to live his life at home. He was able to perform the activities of daily living, but cooking, cleaning and doing laundry were beyond his physical strength and abilities. His family divided up the chores. One daughter lived close by, so she would stop by and check on him every morning and evening. She managed his money and brought his groceries. The other daughter performed weekly housecleaning and laundry duty. Both daughters cooked and brought meals that Raymond could warm in the microwave. Out-of-town daughter would fly in several times a year to give her sisters a respite break and do chores. A grandson mowed the grass and kept the yard tidy. By doing the IADL tasks, Raymond's family performed the chores he could no longer do and enabled him to live at home.

Where can help be found? A telephone call to the local 211 network or Area Agency on Aging starts the caregiving family toward resources available to them. Some families may find resources available that they never expected — some at no cost, others on a sliding scale. Some families will find it necessary to pay for help, but isn't paying for help better than the primary caregiver losing his health?

What does Dad need in terms of care? Is Dad mentally capable but physically in poor health? Is Dad's physical health good but mentally he is slipping? Caregiving families may feel they need help making decisions about living arrangements. What does Dad want? Can family members and friends build a supportive group which provides his needs? Would he sell his house and move in with one of the adult children? Does he want to move to a senior citizen apartment located in town? If he is mentally alert and capable, he should be a part of these decisions.

The AARP resource book, *Caring for your Parents*, provides these statistics:

Who Lives Where

A little over half of care recipients still live in their own homes.
About 20 to 25 percent live in the same household as their caregivers.
About 4 percent of care recipients live in assisted living facilities.
About 5 percent of recipients are in nursing homes.
African Americans and Hispanics are more likely than whites to live in multigenerational households."[4]

Safety Issues for an Elder Person Living at Home

Medical Alert System

Raymond's family signed him up with a medical alert system called Lifeline. This around-the-clock monitored alert system was available through a local hospital. A volunteer came to Raymond's home and installed the console. Raymond and his family learned how to activate a call for help: Raymond pushed the button he wore around his neck. During the sign-up period, the family gave multiple phone numbers (in the order they preferred to be called) in case of emergency.

One day Raymond stepped out his dining room door and onto the deck. His foot slipped and he found himself lying on the wet deck floor. When he pushed his Lifeline button, he wasn't able to talk loud enough for them to hear him. The Lifeline staff immediately called the first family member's phone number. Raymond's daughter left work and went to his home to find her dad lying on the deck. She called for a grandson to help get him back on his feet. Raymond was sore and bruised but had no major injuries. This family was very glad Raymond was wearing his Lifeline button so he could call for help.

People should expect a monthly fee for the medical alert system. Raymond's family felt the Lifeline system was money well spent. It enabled Raymond to call for help when he needed and provided peace of mind for his daughters, who were juggling their jobs as they supported their father's decision to continue living at home.

Preventing Falls

Raymond had fallen several times before but one day he fell into the closet, wiping out the closet door and fracturing his shoulder. While he was in the hospital on the rehabilitation floor, a fall assessment was done and physical therapy was recommended to improve his gait and muscle strength. Raymond worked hard at the therapy because he wanted to go home. His family was amazed at the strength and improved gait he developed in that few weeks of therapy.

"Accidents are the fifth leading cause of death among older adults, with falls ranking first in this category."[5] For people aged 60 and older, falls rank as the number one cause for the eight million fractures which happen worldwide every year. "Falls occur in 30–60% of older adults each year, and 10–20% of these result in injury, hospitalization and/or death."[6]

People fear breaking their hips. Most hip fractures require surgery and months of healing time. For people 75 years and older, hip fractures can require up to a year of recovery time in a nursing home and an increased risk of death from the fracture and its complications. Another commonly occurring fracture involves the wrist. Wrist fractures occur when a person tries to catch himself and falls on his outstretched hand. Such a fracture can require surgery and hardware to hold the broken bones while healing occurs.

Doctors recognize the value of preventing falls and injuries and much research has gone into this complicated topic. Begin fall prevention by eliminating dangers in the home environment. The Foundation for Health in Aging, established by the American Geriatrics Society, provides these suggestions for making home a safer place: Remove loose carpets and rugs and secure rugs or substitute rugs with nonskid backing to help prevent falls. Add lights in dimly lit areas, including the top and bottom of stairs, to illuminate a danger zone. Night-lights in bedrooms, bathrooms and hallways help people see so they can move about safely at night. All clutter, especially near stairs, should be removed to provide a safe walkway. Grab bars in the bathroom, near the toilet and in the tub or shower contributes to safety while a nonslip floor surface in the tub or shower helps prevent slips and falls. Many adults find a tall toilet easier and safer to use. Nonslip shoes will also help prevent falls; socks or loose slippers can cause slips which result in falls.[7]

Other suggested home modifications to improve safety include installing handrails on both sides of stairways, placing barriers at dangerous locations, and removing thresholds to prevent falls. Improved lighting contributes to a safer environment. Installing lighted switch plates and using high-wattage bulbs in hazardous locations increases safety for everyone. Bright, contrasting colors may help the care receiver who has visual problems see where he's going.

To improve accessibility and ease of use, a wheelchair ramp in the garage or to the front door may be needed. Furniture can be rearranged to ensure a pathway wide enough for a walker or a wheelchair. Furniture should fit the person comfortably with the height of their arms and seat to enable the person to stand easily. Get rid of unstable furniture. Lever-type doorknobs and faucets may be easier for arthritic hands to grip. Flexible hand-held shower heads enable a person to control where the water sprays. A properly fitting shower bench allows the care receiver to sit comfortably and safely during showers. Clocks and telephones with large numbers and buttons are easier to use. Easy to use electronics such as single-serving coffee pots may simplify life for the care receiver.

"Most falls are associated with identifiable risk factors, such as weakness, unsteady gait, confusion and psychoactive medications."[8] A fall assessment workup can help a person and his caregivers identify possible causes for falls. Some causes cannot be changed but much progress can be made after a fall assessment. After identifying a person's risk factors for falling, a plan can be made to correct problems. Working with a person's doctor, caregivers can make the environment safer. Medical treatments, including medication adjustments, can help prevent falls.

Wintertime falls happen when Mom decides to go get her morning newspaper on an icy sidewalk. Or she decides she will venture to the mailbox today: "After all, the snow is almost completely melted after yesterday's sunshine."

The American Geriatric Society recommends fall prevention during winter days, including avoiding walking on icy or snowy sidewalks. A dry sidewalk is safer to walk on. Shoes with nonskid soles are safer than slick-soled shoes. Steps and sidewalks should be carefully shoveled by a healthy individual. A good suggestion is to hire someone to shovel sidewalks and steps.[9]

Preventing Fires, Using Smoke Detectors and Carbon Monoxide Detectors

Smoke detectors should be installed and operational — at least one on each floor of the home. Smoke detectors should be located near bedrooms, on the ceiling or 6 to 12 inches below the ceiling on a wall. All electrical outlets and switches should have appropriate cover plates. When a person touches the plastic of an electrical outlet, it should not be hot or unusually warm. If it is, the increased warmth may indicate unsafe wiring. All cords and appliances should then be unplugged and an electrician called to check the wiring and outlet or switch for safety.

All heat sources, space heaters, wood burning heating equipment, and chimneys should be in proper working order with regular cleaning and inspection to prevent fires. "Keep a fire extinguisher that can be used for a variety of types of fires, including chemical fires, in areas where you use fireplaces, wood stoves, and kerosene heaters."[10]

Smoking in bed can cause a fire. "Among mattress and bedding fire-related deaths in a recent year, 42% were to persons 65 and older."[11] Nothing — not blankets, comforters or the family pet — should be on top of an electric blanket when the blanket is turned on. Electric blankets should not be tucked in. No one should sleep with a heating pad turned on as this could cause a burn.

The International Association of Certified Home Inspectors (Inter-NACHI) gives additional suggestions to make a home safer. Prevent burns from hot tap water and open flame. Tap water burns can be prevented by setting the water heater at "low" or below 120 degrees Fahrenheit. The kitchen area, with the stove and oven, is an increased risk for burn injury. Create a fire-free zone around the stove and the oven. Remove towels and other flammables from the stove/oven area. Make sure curtains cannot brush against heat sources and catch fire. The U.S. Consumer Product Safety Commission estimates "that 70% of all people who die from clothing fires are over 65 years of age. Long sleeves are more likely to catch fire than are short sleeves. Long sleeves are also more apt to catch on pot handles, overturning pots and pans and causing scalds." The InterNACHI recommends that you "roll back long, loose sleeves or fasten them with pins or elastic bands while you are cooking."[12] This organization gives a home safety checklist which caregiving families can access at http://www.nachi.org/elderlysafety.htm.

Avoid dangers of electrical and phone cords by arranging furniture so outlets are available and extension cords aren't needed. Cords should never have furniture weight on them, as damage can cause electric shock and fire hazards. Cords should never be placed under carpeting, as a fire might result. Using tape to attach cords to walls is safer than using staples or nails, which could damage the cords and cause a fire or electrical shock. Small electrical appliances, in both the kitchen and the bathroom, should not be located close to water and should be unplugged until needed.

Carbon monoxide poisoning poses a danger when fuels such as wood, natural gas, kerosene and others are used. This invisible gas has no odor and can be lethal. The American Geriatrics Society recommends these actions to avoid carbon monoxide poisoning. Have fireplace chimneys and wood stove flues inspected yearly and cleaned when needed. Install a battery-operated carbon monoxide detector close to fireplaces, wood stoves and kerosene heaters: "Open a window — just a crack will do — when using a kerosene stove."[13] Keep space heaters at least 3 feet away from curtains, bedding, furniture or anything which could catch fire. Use only equipment appropriate for indoor use; don't try to heat the house with a charcoal barbecue grill.

Emergency Preparedness —
What Happens When the Lights Go Out?

Could Mom prevent a heat-related illness when the heat index is through the roof and her air conditioner doesn't work? The risk of heat exhaustion, and the life threatening heatstroke, increases in older people (age 65 and older), whose bodies cannot adjust as easily as those of younger people. Older people may also be taking prescription medications which increase the danger of heat exhaustion or heatstroke.

Preventing heat-related illnesses is the best strategy. When a person recognizes the potential danger of them, he can begin drinking extra fluids before he starts to feel thirsty. By the time a person feels thirsty, he has already lost significant fluids. "Warning: if your physician limits the amount of fluid you drink or has you on water pills, check with him on how much you should drink while the weather is hot."[14] The best choices of liquids to drink include water and slightly salty sports drinks: avoid alcohol, large amounts of sugar and caffeinated drinks, as they can contribute to fluid loss and dehydration.

Other strategies for preventing overheating include wearing lightweight, light-colored, loose-fitting clothing and seeking a cool shelter. If a person's home has a basement, it will be cooler than the upstairs. If a basement isn't available, are there air conditioned public shelters available to the public?

Heat exhaustion results when a person's body loses large amounts of fluids and salt through sweating. The person becomes dehydrated and loses valuable salts through sweating. Symptoms of heat exhaustion include fatigue, nausea, excessive thirst, and weakness. Mental alertness decreases and there may be confusion, anxiety or agitation. The person may become dizzy and faint and may have a headache. The heart rate may become slow or weakened. The person's body continues sweating and tries to cool itself until it runs out of fluids. A person may experience heat cramps, which are severe cramps in the muscles most often used (hands, feet, and calves). These painful muscle cramps may seem to last forever, but are from one to three minutes. The goal of treating heat exhaustion and heat cramps is to replace the lost fluids and salt. When heat exhaustion becomes heatstroke, a person's body can no longer cool itself. Heatstroke becomes a life-threatening situation with soaring body temperatures and a great risk of complications. It requires hospitalization.

WebMD makes this recommendation for the treatment of heat-related illnesses: "Get help. It is critical that emergency medical assistance be called as soon as possible. Then, if possible, get the victim to drink, but don't force fluids if the person is confused or passed out.... Victims should be moved to a cool environment, lie flat or with their feet raised slightly above head level, and sip a cool, slightly salty beverage — such as a salty sports drink, salted tomato juice, cool bouillon, or plain drinking water with salt added (one level teaspoon of salt per quart of water)."[15]

Keeping the Chill Off

Hypothermia (low body temperature) can harm older people. As people age, their metabolism slows down and they may not recognize they are getting too cold. Hypothermia can be fatal to anyone, but older people face an increased danger of death from hypothermia.

Some suggested behaviors to prevent hypothermia include staying dry, wearing multiple thin layers of loose-fitting clothing, staying indoors and minimizing outside activities to preserve body heat. Appropriate outside clothes includes a coat, hat, boots, gloves or mittens and a scarf to cover one's mouth and nose.[16]

One might think a common symptom of hypothermia would be shivering. Shivering does mean that a person is getting cold. However, some older people don't shiver — or not as much as they did in younger years — so shivering may or may not be present in an older person suffering from being too cold. Other symptoms of hypothermia include feeling tired, confused, sleepy, apathetic, weak; cold, pale skin; difficulty walking; diminished breathing or heart rate.

When hypothermia happens, what does one do? Check the unconscious person carefully for breathing and a pulse while dialing 911 for emergency medical personnel. Check for a pulse for at least one minute before beginning cardiopulmonary resuscitation (CPR) because a hypothermic victim's heart rate may be slow and weak.

Rewarming the person is the second priority. If the person is outside, bring him inside to a warm place and replace all wet clothes with dry ones. If the person is awake and able to swallow, give him warm fluids (caffeine or alcohol are not recommended). "Warm the person's body first by wrapping in blankets. Warming hands and feet first can cause shock. Do not immerse him in warm water because rapid warming can cause heart irregularities. If using hot water bottles or chemical hot packs, wrap them in cloth first before using to prevent skin injury."[17] While these first-aid actions are being done, get medical help.

Frostbite occurs when ice crystals form in a person's tissues; it can result in damage to tissues, even to the point of gangrene (death of the tissues). Frostbite most commonly affects the extremities (hands and feet) and the face (nose, ears, cheeks and chin.) One should suspect frostbite when the skin looks "white or ashy (for people with darker skin) or grayish-yellow, skin that feels hard or waxy" or when the body part has lost feeling (numb).[18]

Frostbite can be prevented by staying indoors and keeping warm. If a person must spend time outside, prevent frostbite by covering all parts of the body. Hypothermia prevention strategies such as keeping dry, limiting the time spent outside in cold weather and wearing multiple light layers of clothing help prevent frostbite also.

Treatment for frostbite includes WebMD's advice: While transporting the person with frostbite to medical care, assist him so he does not walk on his frostbitten toes or feet. Also, recognize that a person who has frostbite is probably hypothermic as well and they need medical help. Transport a frostbite or hypothermia victim to a medical facility as quickly as possible for the best chances of recovery. Any constrictive jewelry and clothing should be loosened or removed to prevent blocked blood flow. It's recommended that a frostbite victim (as with a hypothermic victim) drink warm, nonalcoholic, noncaffeinated fluids. A dry, sterile bandage can be placed between the affected fingers and toes to prevent damage from rubbing. Experts do not recommend that a person rub the affected areas as it can cause harm to tissues. Until medical care can be obtained, follow these WebMD suggestions: "Do not rewarm the skin until you can keep it warm. Warming and then reexposing the frostbitten area to cold air can cause worse damage. Gently warm the area in warm water until the skin appears red or warm.... Do not use direct heat from heating pads, radiator, or fire."[19]

Emergency Disaster Plan Begins with Communication

Each caregiving family should develop a plan for emergencies. If a winter ice storm knocked out electrical power, who would assist Dad? Does he have a phone which would work without electricity? By communicating ahead of the disaster, a family can make a plan. Perhaps in-town son should be the first person called when Dad needs help. After Dad is safe, warm and fed, in-town son can call the next person on the family disaster call list with the news and suggestions of what is needed next.

Does Dad have phone numbers readily available? This list should include local family members and trusted neighbors, as well as the police, fire department and local poison control number. This list should be up-to-date, legible, large enough for the person to read easily and placed in multiple locations, including near the phone. Some elderly family members can use their cell phones to summon help. Emergency phone numbers should be added to that phone's contact list.

As part of the emergency plan, the American Geriatric Society's Foundation for Health in Aging recommends these strategies: pick two meeting places in case an evacuation is necessary, one close to home and one outside the neighborhood where family can meet. Make a plan for travel if evacuation is necessary. Who could pick up Dad and drive him to the out-of-neighborhood meeting place? This designated driver should contact the local authorities for their emergency plan and evacuation routes in case of a disaster. This information should be kept in the designated driver's vehicle.

A medical alert ID bracelet would be helpful for a person who has chronic health problems such as diabetes, asthma, Parkinson's disease or epilepsy. These illnesses might complicate the elder person's ability to talk with emergency workers. Valuable information can be engraved on a medic alert bracelet or pendant, such as illnesses, allergies to drugs or foods, any prescribed medications and emergency contacts.

Emergency medical kits would be important during a disaster. A two-week supply of medicines would be valuable during a disaster time. "Since insurance companies usually won't pay for more than a 30-day supply, consider asking your doctor for an extra prescription, and paying for it out-of-pocket. Another option is to fill prescriptions a week early each month until you have at least a 2-week supply for emergencies."[20] Keep these medications in the original packaging. Don't put this 2-week supply on the shelf and let it get old. Always use the older supply of medications and rotate the stock of medication so none become outdated. If medications such as insulin need to be refrigerated, ice packs and an insulated bag will be needed to store the medication properly.

Medical equipment used frequently would need to be included in the emergency medical kit. Equipment such as a blood glucose monitor, batteries for hearing aids, CPAP machine and supplies, etc., would be needed during a disaster. An extra pair of eyeglasses, hearing aid or dentures might be needed. The American Geriatrics Society recommends that a disaster supply kit should include the following items in addition to the emergency medical kit:

- One gallon of water per person per day (supply for a minimum of three days, preferably a two-week supply),
- three-day supply of canned and dried (nonperishable) foods
- basic supplies such as a manual can opener, flashlight, portable radio with extra batteries, knife
- food preparation supplies such as knife, basic cooking utensils, aluminum foil and plastic bags, plates and eating utensils, waterproof matches, trash bags for garbage
- complete change of clothing for each person (including winter clothes such as coat, hat, mitten, scarf, long-sleeved shirts and pants, shoes)
- one blanket for each person
- contact information for family, friends and doctors.
- cash in case the bank ATMs aren't available — the recommended amount is $500 or as close to that amount as possible
- basic hygiene products including soap, toothpaste, toothbrushes, hand sanitizer, toilet paper, sunscreen, baby wipes
- first aid kit or emergency kit.[21]

Protecting Mom or Dad from Scam Artists

Caregiver families may find themselves cleaning up the situation when Mom gives an unknown contractor permission to paint her house. When a contractor stopped at her house, he offered to paint it. Mom thought it sounded like a good idea and agreed to his quote. When she mentioned this project to her son, he became very concerned. When she showed him the quote, her son said, "Mom, this is highway robbery. That's too much money for a paint job. If you want your house painted, we can have it done but not by this company. I've never heard of this company. I need to look into this situation because it looks like a scam." The family began by calling the phone number on the paperwork and telling them that they should not paint the house or contact their mom. They also contacted the attorney general's office and asked for help: was this company legitimate? what should they do to cancel the job (other than that first phone call)?

Consumer fraud can be a huge concern for caregiving families whose loved one still lives at home. The American Bar Association book, *You and Your Aging Parents,* gives valuable details about elder abuse, exploitation and consumer fraud schemes. Highlights of this chapter include this: "Victims of elder abuse can come from any educational background, ethnic background, or economic class.... Elder abuse can come in a number of forms, including: physical, emotion, or sexual abuse; neglect or abandonment by caregivers, which can be either passive or active; and financial exploitation.... If your parent is the victim of elder abuse, first talk to your parent about what options and remedies he or she would like to pursue.... Consumer fraud is more than pushy salespeople; perpetrators of consumer fraud are skilled professional criminals who prey on vulnerable individuals.... Perpetrators of consumer fraud can reach your parents even if you think they are safe.... Your parents can protect themselves from identity theft by being careful about revealing personally identifiable information, not using easily obtainable passwords, and immediately notifying the three national credit-reporting agencies if their wallets go missing."[22]

Caregiving families face many challenges while caring for their loved ones. Planning ahead and utilizing resources available to them can simplify the day-to-day challenges.

9

Grieving and Remembering

Peggy Gross was shocked the morning of August 25, 2010, when she found her husband of 45 years lying unresponsive on the living room floor. She knew her husband, Don, had many health problems, including congestive heart failure, vascular disease, chronic obstructive pulmonary disease and diabetes. There had been times when she expected him to succumb to his illnesses, but not this day.

The previous night had been a good one. Instead of struggling to sleep sitting up in his recliner, he had slept in bed for several hours. At bedtime, he told her he loved her and thanked her for taking good care of him. He said he could not have had a better wife over all their years together. She had checked on him several times through the night and found him sleeping and breathing easily. She was thinking the new medicine for congestive heart failure was working, and she was pleased with this progress.

The next time she got up, around 6 A.M., he wasn't in his bed. She glanced in the living room and saw that he wasn't in his recliner. She walked in and saw him lying on the floor in front of the loveseat. Peggy continues: "I could not find any breathing or get a response. I called 911 and told them he wasn't responding. The police officer showed up first and then the ambulance. They determined it had probably been about an hour since he had passed away. Because he had been feeling better the night before and it was the first night we both got to sleep in bed during the past two weeks, it was a sinking feeling to find him and know that he was gone."[1]

Peggy functioned in a fog the next few days. She had missed so much sleep during the past two weeks that she was physically exhausted: "I had mixed emotions. I was sad for myself, but relieved for him who had been suffering. It deflated me; I couldn't think as clearly as I thought I should. I didn't know what to say. I didn't know how to feel. I don't know how to describe it better." [2]

She remembers the family rallied bringing food, making plans and eventually sitting together and "remembering" Don. She heard some stories for the first time. They planned the funeral service, which included Don's favorite scriptures and hymns. Instead of a single eulogy, each member of the immediate family wrote a paragraph which was read.

Son Greg Gross shared these thoughts in the eulogy: "My dearest dad, I am so sad for us, the ones left behind, but for you I am so happy; no more medicine, no more pain or misery, no more breathing problems. You have always 'been there' for me.... You have been preparing us for this moment for the last 10 years; I now find comfort in your preparation, understand what you were doing and it is making this much easier than it would have been. I love you. You will be missed but never forgotten."[3]

Grandson Michael remembers when he had the privilege of taking Don to a St. Louis Blues hockey game: "I got a chance to see him as a kid again, so full of life and happy in an unhappy time for him. I will never forget the look on his face when they [hockey players] took the ice."[4]

Grandson Keith shared his thoughts: "I am not a person of many words as my grandfather was, but one thing that he did teach me was to always let my opinion be well known. So in my opinion, Don was the best hard headed, stubborn, opinionated, honest, loving, and most active grandpa anyone could ask for. Not to mention the best teacher. He taught me how to drive, shoot, and he taught me how to speak my mind, so all in all he taught me the three most important skills for a good case of road rage." Amid chuckles from the family, the jokester ended with, "I love you, grandpa Don."[5]

Peggy shared these thoughts: "Don was always a person who had an opinion and always made his opinion known and I'm sure he was pleased and flattered. The family found the service to be healing."[6]

Grieving

"Trust that nature will do the healing. Know that the pain will pass, and when it passes, you will be stronger, happier, more sensitive and aware."[7] People grieve when significant people in their lives die. The death of a stranger won't bring about a significant feeling or behaviors of loss; people grieve for those with whom they share a bond.

British psychiatrist John Bowlby explained a basic human need for security and safety in terms of "attachment." At an early age, children form an attachment to parents and significant others. These attachments develop "early in life, are usually directed toward a few specific individuals, and tend to endure throughout a large part of the life cycle." As children grow and mature, they venture out and experience the world but they always return to the significant people to whom they are "attached" for support and safety. "When the attachment figure disappeared or is threatened, the response is one of intense anxiety and strong emotional protest."[8]

Scientists have observed similar behaviors in the animal world when a mate disappears and the animal grieves. One example given occurred at the Montreal zoo: "After one of the dolphins died, its mate refused to eat, and the zookeepers had the difficult, if not impossible, task of keeping the surviving dolphin alive. By not eating, the dolphin was exhibiting manifestations of grief and depression akin to human loss behavior."[9]

Grief involves physical manifestations which people commonly experience after a loss of a person to whom they're attached. Physical characteristics (or symptoms) of normal grief include bodily distresses such as a tight feeling in the chest or throat, a hollow feeling in the stomach, dry mouth, feeling exhausted or short of breath and lacking energy. Some people will be fearful they won't remember what their loved one looked like and will become preoccupied. Others deal with feelings of hostility and feelings of being unable to function.[10]

People who are grieving may find themselves unable to sleep. Some will find themselves preoccupied and unable to focus. Appetite disturbances may affect a person. Having no appetite for food is most common but some people may react by overeating. Someone grieving may withdraw socially, feeling it's too much effort to socialize. Some dream of the deceased loved one. One person will hang onto their loved one's belongings and consider them treasures. For someone else, seeing the loved one's belongings may bring pain, so that person may avoid dealing with the belongings.

Grieving also involves emotions. The most common feeling is sadness. Most people feel sad when they've lost a loved one whether or not they shed tears. Many people deal with anger, either because they couldn't prevent the death or because the deceased has left them behind. "In the loss of any important person there is a tendency to regress, to feel helpless, to feel unable to exist without the person, and then to experience the anger that goes along with these feelings of anxiety."[11]

Many caregivers find themselves feeling guilty. They wish they had done more to help Dad or wish they had done things differently. They may believe their efforts weren't enough and blame themselves. To live in the moment, the caregivers should forgive self and not mourn for what they cannot change. They should recognize that human beings aren't perfect and human efforts won't be perfect. Caregivers freed from regrets will be able to live wisely in the present.

A grieving wife may feel anxiety: "How can I survive without him? I cannot take care of this house and yard by myself. What am I to do?" One woman received wise advice from her lawyer to not make any major changes for one year. She hired help from a neighborhood boy, who mowed her grass and did chores she could not manage. Eighteen months later she told her lawyer he had given her good advice: she now realized she could continue living in her home. She dealt with her anxiety in a constructive way and gained confidence in her ability to cope. "Carried to extremes, this anxiety can develop into a full-blown phobia."[12]

Grieving family members may deal with feelings of loneliness, helplessness, shock, yearning for the loved one, and numbness. When the loved one suffers through a lingering illness, caregivers may have already traveled through the grief and find they feel relief and freedom from the load of caring for Dad. "If grief is defined as one's experiences after a loss, then mourning is the process one goes through leading to an adaptation to the loss."[13]

Four Tasks of the Bereaved (J. William Worden)

The first is "to accept reality of loss.... The first task of grieving is to come full face with the reality that the person is dead, that the person is gone and will not return."[14]

The ritual of a funeral or memorial service can help family members accept the new reality. Don's family honored him when each person wrote memories of his effect on their lives. These memories were shared at the funeral service and brought tears and chuckles as the family celebrated their loved one's life.

Different religions have different services they perform. Funerals and memorial services can bring closure and comfort to grieving family members and friends as they work through their sorrow. This ritual is only the first step in the journey of grief; the grieving process takes time and involves both emotional and intellectual acceptance.

The second task is "to work through the pain of grief ... the literal physical pain that many people experience and the emotional and behavioral pain associated with loss." Dr. Worden states "it is impossible to lose someone you have been deeply attached to without experiencing some level of pain."[15]

Third is "to adjust to an environment in which the deceased is missing.... [T]here are three areas of adjustment that one needs to make after losing a loved one to death. There are external adjustments — how the death affects one's everyday functioning in the world, internal adjustments — how the death affects one's sense of self, and spiritual adjustments — how the death affects one's beliefs, values and assumptions about the world."[16] Several months after Don's death, Peggy called and asked her sister to come help clean out her husband's closet, saying, "I just can't get started at cleaning out his things. Will you come help me?"[17] Having a supportive helper made it easier. The two women worked together to box up those belongings: some were saved in the garage, others were donated and the worn out things were thrown away. Internal adjustments include feeling vulnerable: "Can I make it without him? I don't know how to drive a car. I've never managed our finances. How can I survive without him?" This widow needs to give herself time to heal and get supportive help from trusted loved ones who can help her manage and gain confidence that she can cope with her new reality.

The fourth and last task is "to emotionally relocate the deceased and move on with life.... [W]e need to find ways to memorialize, that is, to remember the dead loved one — keeping them with us but still going on with life."[18] A gravesite and tombstone has served this purpose for many years. One woman finds herself traveling to her parents' gravesite every Mother's Day, a journey that brings her peace and comfort deep inside.

People must travel through the stages of grief and accomplish these tasks to get past the sorrow and grief of losing their loved one. These stages and tasks have been likened to a "lightning bolt, full of ups and downs, progressions and regressions, dramatic leaps and depressing backslides. Realize this and know that whether you are 'better' or 'worse' than yesterday — or five minutes ago — the healing process is underway."[19] Some suggestions for how to handle grief include these:

"Don't expect the process to be easy or impossible; avoid both extremes.
Don't compare the time it takes you with the time it has taken someone else.

Draw on your preexisting support structures, that being your family, friends, and family of faith in church.

Deal with issues, don't avoid them. Despite the temptation to give up or at least procrastinate, move ahead with necessary actions.

Deal with belongings; avoid extremes. Don't just give everything away, keep what is special. But don't create "shrines."

Expect unusual emotions. You may experience confusion more than ever before. Often people speak of feeling a weight upon their shoulders or their chest, holding them back.

When you feel a good cry coming on, make it a positive experience by reflecting upon good memories.

Think through and plan for holidays, birthdays, anniversaries, and the like."[20]

Supportive Friends Can Help During Grieving

Peggy's best friend called to say she wanted to prepare the funeral day meal. This woman and her husband prepared and served a feast after the funeral to the 40 family members and close friends. It wasn't until later that Peggy learned her friend prepared the meal in spite of a broken toe. Two days before the funeral the friend had dropped a large can of vegetables on her foot. She swore her husband to secrecy because she wanted to prepare the funeral meal for this family. The woman showed her compassion and love to a grieving family and helped them carry their sorrow. Other friends brought food such as fresh lunch meat and a red velvet cake the family enjoyed. Friends stopped by to visit, showing their love and support. Upon her return to work, Peggy was touched by her many coworkers who stopped by to give a hug and warm words of comfort.

Caring friends can listen to the grieving family members when they need someone to listen. A friend can sit quietly and offer a shoulder to cry on and lean on. They don't need magic words but rather a sensitive heart and sincere caring to help the grieving person carry the load. One woman's father had died on her birthday. During a conversation with her best friend, she said it hurt to always think of her father's death on her birthday. They agreed they would move her birthday celebration to the week prior the birthday.

Anticipatory Grief

Anticipatory grief means "grieving that occurs prior to the actual loss."[21] Peggy says, "In 2000 Don was so sick before the doctors recognized it was his heart and did surgery, none of us thought he was going to make it. There was a lot of grieving done by the whole family. But then he recovered from the surgery, got better and life went on."[22]

Some caregivers may find themselves grieving early, before Mom dies. A family may begin to grieve the loss of their mother as they watch her lose touch with reality. They feel pain when she no longer recognizes their faces or can call them by name. They grieve as they force themselves to go visit her in the Alzheimer's unit. They sit with her and talk about the weather, repeating the same sentence every visit. While she does not call them by name, she seems to know they are significant people to her and she stops walking in her geri-chair and sits with them. They visit, take care of her clothes, and bring supplies she needs because it's the right thing to do. These families may travel through anticipatory grief long before Mom's death. Some families may still deal with grief after the death, but some may have dealt with it beforehand.

Psychologists recognize that the person who is dying may experience anticipatory grief. The older person who is mentally capable may recognize his time to live is short: "The person who is dying often has many attachments in his own life and, to that extent, will be losing many significant others all at once."[23]

Don worked to prepare his family for his death, Peggy recalls:

> I remember Don commenting that when his younger brother found out he had cancer at age 31, this brother was concerned about how his family would cope with his death. That describes Don well. Don was concerned about how his family, especially his son Greg and grandsons Michael and Keith, would feel about his death. They handled it extremely well and it's because of Don's preparation. Don would say things like "I will be fine; I will get to see my parents and brother" and "Don't be sad for me." He told Peggy "You can do that project on the house after I'm gone" and "Have your little pity party then move on with life." Don's preparation was a key in all our healing process. It's amazing how well the whole family has adjusted and his preparing us is the reason.[24]

Parents who are losing their young child to a terminal illness may experience anticipatory grieving. "When one loses a child there is the sense of untimeliness about the death. Children are not supposed to die before their parents — it is not in the natural order of things."[25]

Sudden Death

Sudden death occurs without warning and can result from heart attacks, accidental deaths and violent deaths such as murder. Sudden death pounces on the family and is a major shock and a painful event. The family and friends grapple to deal with the loss of a loved one snatched from their lives: "Sudden deaths are often more difficult to grieve than other deaths in which there is some prior warning that death is imminent."[26]

Dr. Worden says survivors of sudden death may feel like they're in a daze and can't come to grips. This feeling may persist for a long time and be accompanied by nightmares. Survivors may feel guilt. They may think "if only I had been there." Or they may need to blame someone or something. They may feel anger at someone, whether it's the person who caused the accident, the person who murdered their loved one or God. Survivors of sudden death deal with unfinished details. They wish they had said "I love you" the last time they saw their loved one, or they wish they had made one more trip to a "special" locale. Survivors of sudden death may feel helpless. Because these survivors had no warning of the death, they may find themselves struggling. They should not compare themselves with others' experiences, as each situation is different and each family deals with grief in their own way and own timing.

Survivors of sudden death can find comfort from loving family and friends as they wade through the shock, pain and sorrow. They need to travel the steps to healing, along with all those who grieve their family member's death. Some survivors will find they need counseling to deal with their loss, and they should get the help they need to deal constructively with it.

Elderly People Grieve

"I've buried so many people I love: Mama and Papa, my brothers and sisters and many old friends. It's hard giving up so many people I've loved." Rebecca voiced the sorrow she felt. Because she had lived a long life, she had lost many people she loved. People age and their circle of family and friends becomes smaller. For some older people, their health becomes a limiting factor and they cannot get out to socialize and make new friends. These people find themselves very limited physically and socially. Grieving can be difficult for sick, elderly people.

Depression

Caregiving can be depressing and exhausting. Researchers found that from 6 percent to 50 percent of caregivers find themselves feeling depressed.[27] Some people call it "situational depression" when dealing with the illness and death of a loved one causes caregivers to feel down and depressed. Situational depression is usually triggered by an outside stress and generally goes away when the person has adjusted or when the stress has resolved itself. Its symptoms include feelings of hopelessness and sadness, frequent crying, anxiety, worry, changes in appetite (either overeating or loss of appetite), sleep problems, headaches, lack of energy and palpitations.[28]

When a caregiver begins to feel overwhelmed or exhausted by his caregiving duties, he should see his doctor and talk about taking care of self. This caregiver may find that antidepressant medications and a support group for caregivers who understand what he's dealing with daily are a tremendous help. Some individuals may need psychotherapy counseling.

Research has shown "that care giving is not only potentially depressing but consuming. The longer you give your all for a loved one, the less you may seem able to make time for your own needs. Life shrinks down to a narrow focus on getting through the day's feeding, toileting and pill doling. Self-neglect breeds social isolation when you stop responding to friends' overtures. It is not unusual for caregivers to forgo medical care for themselves, even though they may be visiting doctors weekly with their loved one. This puts you at risk for unwittingly sacrificing your own physical health."[29]

Peggy worried about whether Don's health would deteriorate to the point that she would need to retire early and care for him. She knew her job kept her in touch with the world outside her home. She wanted to work two more years before she retired for financial reasons, but she wasn't sure what to do. She worried about Don and his health; if it declined more, she was going to have to quit working and care for him. When he passed away, the family recognized she would not have to make that decision.

Significant Days Cause Grieving Pain

Anniversaries and significant days can plunge a person back into the grieving process. The first Valentine's Day, the first birthday, wedding anniversary and other significant days can trigger a person's memories and bring pain and grieving back into their thoughts.

Peggy shared these thoughts six months after Don's death:

> I have found myself in a real funk this week.... I've been irritable and tears have come easily. This week I've faced Valentine's Day alone. Don's birthday is coming up and it has been six years since Mother died. I've talked to myself all week ... but it's been a challenge. Guess I can't expect it to go smoothly all the time.... The easiest way I have found to cope ... is to recognize what the event is, have a short pity party for me, remember the good things and when the day is past, things return to normal until the next one comes along. As time goes on, I seem to recognize the source of my "funk" more quickly and it is helping make the process go more smoothly dealing with my parent's deaths. I expect it to be the same with Don's death.[20]

Other family members are dealing with Don's death. Son Greg says this:

> Not a day goes by that I don't think about Dad and miss him.... I seem to be thinking about him a lot this week, probably because Dad's birthday is coming up soon. Grandson Michael mentioned he was having trouble this week, missing Don even more than usual because Nascar is starting and he and Don both followed Nascar as well as Blue's hockey. This will be his first year to not be able to talk to Don about these events. Grandson Keith has found comfort by wearing Grandpa Don's shirts. When asked about it, Keith said wearing one of Don's shirts makes him feel good.[31]

Surviving the Grief by Caring for Self — Physically, Emotionally and Spiritually

A caregiver may find himself grieving at a time when he is exhausted from the physical care of the loved one. He should go back to the basics: care for physical self by getting extra rest, eating healthy foods and drinking adequate amounts of water. "Be gentle with yourself. Don't rush about. Your body needs energy for repair."[32] As he gets rested, this person should begin moderate exercise, which will add energy and conditioning to his physical body. One person may want to go for a walk, while another person may want to do yoga or stretching exercises.

A caregiver can care for self emotionally: "Don't postpone, deny, cover or run from your pain. Be with it. Now. Everything else can wait. An emotional wound requires the same priority treatment as a physical wound. Set time aside to mourn. The sooner you allow yourself to be with your pain, the sooner it will pass. The only way *out* is *through*."[33] The authors of *How to Survive the Loss of a Love* continue: "Be kind to yourself. Stay away from toxic things, situations and people. Take your time. Don't try to understand, comprehend or figure everything out."[34]

A caregiver can care for self spiritually: "Whenever you think of it, ask that you be surrounded by all the Goodness and Light you can imagine." Good is such an obvious thing, it's difficult to define. We all know what we consider the best, the highest, the greatest, the best. You can think of "good" as in *The Good Earth*, or "good" as "God" with an extra "o" added. Light is a concept that seems to permeate almost every religious belief and spiritual practice, from the light of nature to the light of the Holy Spirit and the light of the sun to the light of the Son."[35]

A person dealing with grief should be patient with self and give time to heal. Some individuals will find writing in a journal helpful. Another person will enjoy meditation or prayer. A third person may find healing through laughter. "Humor can give a sense of hope, which provides us with a powerful message that in spite of the loss, all is *not* lost. Life can and does go on."[36] Writer Garrison Keillor expressed it well: "They say such nice things about people at their funerals. It is a shame that I am going to miss mine by only a few days."[37]

With time, the individual who is successfully dealing with grief will find himself feeling more optimistic and alive. His thinking will become clearer and his concentration will improve, and he will find himself interested in being with other people and doing more for other people. He will be more interested in life and things around him. "Loving once and learning to grieve and fully mourn the loss of that love is a good indicator of being able to love again. We cannot just put that earlier love aside, though. It has played a significant role in us evolving in the person we are today. We tuck that love inside us, with all its teachings, and carry it tenderly as we turn to face what life is bringing on."[38]

Eight months after Don's death, Peggy had this to say:

> The memory of Don's voice guides me to do this or not that. One day I hit the curb and damaged a tire. At first I didn't know what to do, and then I thought to myself, "Don would say do this." And that's what I proceeded to do and got it fixed. He was very protective and he always warned me, "Don't put yourself in a dangerous situation. Think about what you're doing and keep yourself safe." He didn't want me to be afraid, but rather to be cautious and aware of my surroundings. If I was meeting a friend for supper and would be going home after dark, I would call and let him know what road I would be traveling in case he would need to come looking for me. The memory of Don's voice makes me feel he's still with me in a good way.[39]

As caregivers and families deal with the end-of-life issues, they should not compare their situation to others and be critical of themselves. Each circumstance is unique and the people involved should be kind to themselves as they cope with the losses of loved ones.

10

Strategies for Healthy Aging

"As with a car, you'll get a lot more mileage out of your body if you perform routine maintenance. Aging is essentially a process in which your cells lose their resilience; they lost their ability to repair damage because the thing you might never have heard of (until now), like mitochondria and telomeres, aren't working the way they should. But it's within your power to boost that resilience and keep your vehicle going an extra couple hundred thousand miles."[1]

The topic of aging and memory loss scares many people. Young healthy people may not worry, but in time everyone dreads the prospects of not remembering what they did yesterday. These individuals wonder if the lost car keys are normal events or if this predicts dire problems. An individual who is watching his mother's mental and physical decline shudders to think what his future holds. Can we prevent or delay memory loss? What can we do to better our chances?

After focusing on 20,000 nurses age 70 and over for several years, researchers at the Nurses' Health Study shared their conclusions in their 2007 newsletter: physical activity, controlled insulin levels, vegetable consumption, maintaining a healthy weight and getting a good night's sleep all contribute to retaining a healthy memory.[2]

A man wonders if he will have a heart attack before age 50 like his father did. Can he do anything to prevent having a heart attack? There's no question a person's genetics affect his health. Genetics, gender and increasing age are three risk factors this man cannot change. However, doctors believe there are healthy lifestyle behaviors people can use to decrease their chances of a heart attack.

The American Heart Association teaches that someone who practices healthy lifestyle habits can change or decrease risk factors, risk factors such as tobacco smoking, high blood pressure, high cholesterol, being physically inactive, being overweight, and having diabetes mellitus. A poor diet, alcohol abuse and not dealing well with stress also can contribute to heart disease.

How does a person age in a healthy manner? Some recommendations include exercise both mentally and physically, controlling blood pressure and cholesterol, controlling insulin levels, consuming a healthy diet with more vegetables and fruits, maintaining a healthy physical weight, getting a good night's sleep, and preventing periodontal disease.

Exercise Your Brain

What can a person do to prevent mental aging? "Stretch your mind — be it through crosswords, Scrabble, chess, or learning how to speak Chinese (if you don't already).... Teaching can save your brain. You're more likely to retain information if you have to explain it to somebody else.... [Y]our brain has a fighting chance if you keep it active and engaged, if you keep challenging it with new lessons, if you learn a new game or new hobby or new vocation."[3]

A healthy cardiovascular system means a healthy blood supply to the brain as well as the body. This means one is less likely to die from a stroke or a heart attack. Experts also believe a healthier brain may delay or prevent memory loss. Healthy behaviors which are good for a person's heart and vascular system contribute to a healthy blood supply to the brain.

Harvard researchers found that "elderly people in the U.S. who have an active social life may have a slower rate of memory decline."[4] Many people recognize that friendships and loving relationships contribute much to a person's well-being and health. Those who are lonely and alone could benefit from volunteering — at their local hospitals, libraries, or schools. Charitable organizations often need volunteers to help achieve their goals. The volunteer would gain social interaction and the organization would gain another pair of helping hands.

Exercise Your Body

The Nurses' Health Study researchers noted that "the more women walked during their late 50s and 60s, the better their memory was at age 70 and older." Walking 90 minutes or more per week resulted in improved cognitive function similar to women eighteen months younger.[5] Increased blood flow to the brain seems to explain (at least partially) why exercise helps retain memory.

Researchers at King's College in London propose an explanation as to why exercise helps keep people young. Professor Tim Spector and Dr. Lynn Cherkas from King's College and Professor Abraham Aviv in New Jersey recruited 2401 volunteers ages 18 to 81 from the United Kingdom. When these researchers looked at the volunteers' DNA they found a difference in telomeres among people who exercised and those who did not exercise. What are telomeres? Telomeres "cap the end of chromosomes in our cells and protect them from damage." Telomeres of sedentary people were found to be shorter than telomeres of people who exercised. Other lifestyle factors these researchers believe shorten the DNA telomeres include obesity and smoking. Both identical and fraternal twins were included in the study. Comparing their telomere length, researchers found that the telomeres of the twin who exercised were "significantly longer" than those of the twin who did not. This was found to be the case in each set of twins. Dr. Cherkas explains: "Overall, the difference in telomere length between the most active subjects and the inactive subjects corresponds to around nine years of aging."[6]

Does a person's stress level affect his telomeres? Yes. Scientists found that mothers dealing with their chronically ill children over a long time (years) had shortened telomeres.[7] Logical thinking would suggest that caregivers dealing with chronic stress might find themselves in a similar situation. What behaviors can caregivers use to deal constructively with their stress? Can exercise decrease a person's stress level? Many people say yes.

Does a sedentary lifestyle increase the risk for inflammation, cell damage and aging? Researchers don't have all the answers. However, they recommend exercise to help keep people healthier and younger. Current recommendations from the Centers for Disease Control and Prevention urge 30 minutes or more of moderate exercise, five or more days a week, plus two days of weight-training. (To access recommendations, see http://www.cdc.gov/physicalactivity/everyone/guidelines/index.html.) This recommendation can easily be broken up into smaller increments of time; even 10-minute segments, which can more easily be fitted into busy schedules. People can choose what type of exercise in which they want to participate. For people concerned with protecting their joints, aerobic exercises recommended by the Arthritis Foundation as being gentle to joints include walking, bicycling and swimming.[8]

Researchers reported findings from the Women's Health Study: "Women who walked two or more hours a week, or who usually walk at a brisk pace (3 mph or faster), had a significantly lower risk of stroke than women who didn't walk."[9]

Keeping Blood Pressure Within Normal Levels

What is blood pressure? Blood pressure reflects the force needed to move blood through the body's arteries. An example of a blood pressure reading is 120/80. The systolic number of 120 shows the heart at work (the amount of blood pushed out of the ventricles of the heart into the aorta, which carries the blood up to the head and down to the rest of the body and the pulmonary artery which carries blood to the lungs). The diastolic number of 80 shows the heart at rest (the aortic valve closes and the blood reloads into the heart chambers ready for the next contraction.)

A blood pressure reading is easily obtained. Medical staff can use a blood pressure cuff and a stethoscope to measure blood pressure. The cuff is wrapped around the upper arm, and the nurse or doctor pumps the small bulb attached to the blood pressure cuff and occludes the blood flow. Then that person listens with a stethoscope against an artery (usually at the inside of elbow) to hear when the sound begins (systolic number) and when the sound ends (diastolic number). Automated blood pressure equipment is also available.

"Normal" blood pressure is defined as a blood pressure reading below 120/80. That means the systolic blood pressure should be below 120 and the diastolic blood pressure below 80. Some fortunate people have a blood pressure reading of 90/60; those individuals should be cheering for their good fortune.

A blood pressure reading is called "prehypertension" when the systolic number is in the 120 to 139 range and the diastolic number is 80–89. A person with prehypertension is considered at risk for developing hypertension. That person's doctor will probably talk about monitoring the blood pressure, some preventive actions a person can take and the possibility of high blood pressure medicine.

When a person's blood pressure is above 140 for the systolic number and 90 for the diastolic number, that person has "hypertension," or high blood pressure. High blood pressure or hypertension "is probably the most common of all health problems in adults and is the leading risk factor for cardiovascular disorders. It affects approximately 50 million individuals in the United States and approximately 1 billion worldwide."[10] Those considered at risk for developing high blood pressure includes anyone with a family history of it. As a person ages, the risk of developing high blood pressure increases. Following menopause women face an increased risk of high blood pressure. As a group, black people deal with higher rates of hypertension than Caucasians.

High blood pressure, if not controlled, does damage quietly to the heart, blood vessels and kidneys and can cause strokes, heart failure and other health problems. Once a person is diagnosed with high blood pressure, he should stay on medication unless his doctor directs otherwise. One should never discontinue high blood pressure medicine on his own.

What causes high blood pressure? A person cannot change some causes of high blood pressure such as genetics, race and age. However, lifestyle causes for high blood pressure — such as high salt intake, eating too much and being overweight or obese, and drinking too much alcohol — can be improved.

High salt intake is believed to contribute to high blood pressure. "At present, salt intake among adults in the United States and United Kingdom averages at least 9 grams/day, with large numbers of people consuming 12 g/day or more. This is far in excess of the maximal intake of 6 g/day for adults recommended by the American Heart Association."[11] Most of the salt intake (6 grams equals a teaspoon of table salt) comes from processed and manufactured foods.

Recommended ways to reduce salt intake is to buy fresh, frozen or "no salt added" vegetables and cook fresh meat and fish instead of processed meats. Herbs and spices can improve the flavor of foods cooked without salt. Rice and pasta should be cooked in water without salt. Reading labels on food packages can help a person decrease the amount of salt he gets from packaged foods. Many restaurants have nutritional information posted on their Internet sites so consumers can check salt levels.

"Drinking too much alcohol can raise blood pressure. It also can harm the liver, brain and heart.... If you drink alcoholic beverages, drink only a moderate amount — one drink a day for women, two drinks a day for men." A drink is defined as 12 ounces of beer, 5 ounces of wine or 1½ ounces of 80 proof whiskey.[12]

Treatments for high blood pressure begin with lifestyle. An overweight person can often decrease his blood pressure as he loses weight. A person who eats a lot of salt can decrease his salt intake and often lower his blood pressure. High blood pressure medications (antihypertensives) can be very successful in controlling blood pressure. There are different types of prescription medicines which treat high blood pressure; they work in different ways. A person should work with his health care provider to control his blood pressure.

Blood Cholesterol Should Be Within Normal Limits

Words like triglycerides and cholesterol are commonly heard terms. What do they mean? Cholesterol is a steroid substance which is essential to the body for formation of bile (which breaks down fats in the diet), manufacture of necessary hormones, and energy metabolism. Triglycerides are the stored form of excess food a person eats and the body doesn't need. These excess calories are turned into triglycerides and stored in fat cells until the body needs them as an energy source. So while cholesterol and fats are necessary for a healthy body, many Americans have elevated levels.

Both cholesterol and triglycerides need transportation through the bloodstream. This transportation involves lipoproteins, which include LDL (low density lipoprotein, or bad cholesterol) and HDL (high density lipoprotein, or good cholesterol). These lipoprotein carriers are produced in both the small intestine and the liver, which explains the genetic factor in cholesterol. Diet alone cannot control a person's cholesterol level if his genes dictate high levels of cholesterol.

LDL carries cholesterol out from the liver to cells, which use the cholesterol to repair the cell membrane and make hormones the body needs. Normal levels of LDL are desirable, and high levels of LDL usually indicate an increased risk of heart disease. HDL carries cholesterol from the body back to the liver, where the body gets rid of it through the bile.

Doctors routinely check blood levels called lipid panels (cholesterol, triglyceride and lipoprotein levels) for their patients. This involves having blood drawn and sent to a lab for testing. The following information is from *Pathophysiology: Concepts of Altered Health States*:

- Total cholesterol levels should be below 200. A number of 200–239 is considered borderline high and a level above 240 is high.

- Triglyceride levels should be below 150 mg/dL. Borderline high levels are 150–199 mg/dL. High levels are 200–499 mg/dL. Very high levels are 500 mg/dL or above.
- HDL, or "good cholesterol" should be above 40, which is considered low. A high number (60 or above) is desired. Doctors believe that regular exercise, controlling the amount of alcohol a person drinks and some lipid medications help elevate the HDL.
- LDL, or "bad cholesterol," blood levels are considered optimal at or below 100 mg/dL. LDL blood levels 100–129 are called near optimal or slightly high. LDL blood levels 130–159 are borderline high. LDL blood levels 160–189 are high. LDL blood levels of 190 are very high.[13]

When a person's lipid panel (blood test) shows a high cholesterol number, high levels of LDL cholesterol and low levels of HDL cholesterol, a person's doctor will begin talking about some changes to correct this situation. Many people have an inherited tendency to high cholesterol (called hypercholesterolemia). The genetics can't be changed. However, dietary and lifestyle changes can help correct the atherosclerosis or hardening of the arteries which can damage a person's heart, blood vessels and organs.

Dietary changes involve decreasing how much a person eats (calorie intake) and what foods he eats. Excess calories contribute to high cholesterol numbers. Saturated fats (animal) and trans fats also contribute to the problem. Trans fats, manufactured from vegetable oils, extend the shelf life of fast foods and enhance their flavor. However, experts recommend that a person eat more fruits, vegetables and fish and less fats, sugar and alcohol and salt.

Lipid-lowering drugs may be prescribed by one's doctor to help lower cholesterol levels, and at least five types of lipid-lowering drugs are available for this purpose. A person should talk to his doctor and pharmacist for details about the drug he receives.

Controlled Insulin Levels

The Nurses' Health Study found that "women with diabetes had worse cognitive function, but that adequate control of the diabetes seemed to help."[14] These researchers speculate that increased blood sugar levels cause problems for the entire body, including the heart and possibly the brain. For more information about diabetes, see chapter 14.

Vegetable Consumption

Women who ate cruciferous vegetables (broccoli, cauliflower, bok choy, and cabbage among others) and green leafy vegetables regularly were found to have cognitive function (thinking, judgment and knowledge) similar to that of women 1 to 2 years younger than they. The more vegetables women ate in their 50s and 60s, the less likely they were to experience memory loss in their 70s and beyond."[15]

Many people do not eat the daily recommended five to nine servings of vegetables and fruits. "Many fruits and vegetables — specifically red grapes, cranberries, tomatoes, onions and tomato juice — contain powerful antioxidants called flavonoids and carotenoids. Found in colorful foods, flavonoids and carotenoids are vitamin-like nonessential substances that seem to decrease inflammation by handcuffing those damaging oxygen free radicals and stimulating your body to take them out of your system through urine."[16] When adding vegetables and fruits into his diet, a person should think colorful foods. There are many colorful vegetables and fruits, from the green of avocadoes, kiwis and broccoli to the yellow of carrots and peppers. For red foods, a person can eat tomatoes, and radishes, while purple foods can be found in eggplants and purple onions.

A healthy diet includes fruits and vegetables, whole grains, fat-free or low-fat milk and milk products, lean meats, poultry, fish, beans, eggs and nuts and is low in saturated fats, trans fats, cholesterol, salt and added sugars. More information can be obtained at the U.S. Department of Agriculture program, "My Plate," at http://www.choosemyplate.gov/tips resources/.

Maintaining a Healthy Physical Weight

Sixty-seven percent of American adults are overweight (32.7 percent) or obese (34.3 percent) according to the United States National Centers for Health Statistics.[17] If maintaining a healthy physical weight were easy, obviously American statistics would be better. Researchers at the RAND Corporation offer new insight: eating should be considered an automatic behavior. If eating is an automatic behavior, proposed approaches include "reducing portion sizes, limiting access to ready-to-eat foods, limiting access to snack foods in schools and workplaces, and reducing food advertising."[18]

Getting a Good Night's Sleep

Kids fight it and adults yearn for it: a good night's sleep. The Nurses' Health Study found that lack of sleep resulted in exhaustion, impaired thinking and poor memory: "Women who typically slept less than 6 hours a night had cognitive function scores similar to those of women 5 years older than them."[19]

Sleep refreshes the mind and body, and animal studies show it is vital to health. Rats normally live two to three years. Rats deprived of rapid eye movement (REM) sleep survive an average of only 5 weeks, while rats deprived of all sleep die within three to four weeks. These rats' immune systems became impaired, and the rats became hypothermic (below normal body temperature) and developed sores on their bodies. Experts suggest that sleep gives neurons in the human brain time to rest and repair. Lack of sleep overloads the neurons; they become depleted in energy and may begin to malfunction. Yet many people struggle to get a good night's sleep.

Two body systems regulate our sleep—the circadian biologic clock and the sleep-wake process. The circadian biologic clock is the body rhythm based on a 24-hour time frame and it's affected by sunlight. The hormone melatonin, which promotes sleep, is regulated by this rhythm. People who must stay awake and work during the nighttime are fighting this biologic clock. The sleep-wake process involves the amount of time a person sleeps versus the amount of time he's awake.

How much sleep does one need? Infants need 16 hours a day and teenagers need an average of 9 hours. Most adults need an average of 7 to 8 hours of sleep. As people age, the sleep requirements may not change but the quality of sleep becomes a problem for some. What can a person do to improve his ability to sleep? The National Sleep Foundation gives these suggestions: "set a schedule ... exercise ... avoid caffeine, nicotine and alcohol ... relax before bed ... sleep until sunlight ... don't lie in bed awake ... control your room temperature ... see a doctor if your sleeping problem continues."[20]

Sleep Apnea

Sleep apnea causes increased risk of stroke. Researchers involved with the Sleep Heart Health Study studied 5422 person age 40 and older and followed them for nine years. At the beginning of the study each participant was evaluated for sleep apnea. Over the nine years, 193 participants had a stroke. Both men and women had increased risk of stroke linked to their sleep apnea. However, men with even mild sleep apnea had increased risk of a stroke and their risk increased with the severity of the sleep apnea. Women faced increased risk of a stroke when they had severe levels of sleep apnea but not mild levels of sleep apnea. [21]

What is sleep apnea? When sleep apnea occurs, the person does not breathe for a brief period of time. These times of not breathing may occur several times during a night's sleep. The most common type of sleep apnea is called obstructive sleep apnea. During sleep, the person's soft tissue in the throat relaxes and blocks the airway. The person's brain arouses them to resume breathing, but their sleep is often of poor quality and results in that person feeling tired and exhausted. Sleep apnea affects more than 12 million Americans and contributes to the development of high blood pressure, memory problems, headaches and cardiovascular disease.

People at risk for sleep apnea include those with a "family history of sleep apnea, excess weight, a large neck, a recessed chin, male sex, abnormalities in the structure of the upper airway, ethnicity (African Americans, Pacific Islanders, and Mexicans), smoking, and alcohol use. Yet sleep apnea can affect both males and females of all ages, including children, and any weight."[22]

Symptoms of sleep apnea include loud snoring and excessive daytime sleepiness and exhaustion. Diagnosis of sleep apnea often occurs after a person spends a night having a sleep study. The most effective treatment for sleep apnea involves a breathing device such as CPAP (continuous positive airway pressure) machine. Surgery to enlarge the airway can also be done. Losing weight may help overweight people with sleep apnea by eliminating extra fat tissue around the neck.[23] More information about sleep apnea and treatments can be found at the American Sleep Apnea Association at http://www.sleepapnea.org/.

Healthy Gums Protect a Person's Heart

Researchers believe they have found a link between periodontal disease (bacteria causing infection of the gums and teeth) and hardening of the arteries. Research done in Austria and Texas evaluated 466 patients who had coronary angioplasty done. Of those 466, 349 patients had coronary heart disease. Of those patients 55.6 percent also had periodontal disease (severe gingivitis) compared to 41 percent of the patients with heart disease but no periodontal disease. The researchers indicated that "periodontal disease represents a potentially modifiable risk factor that is both preventable and treatable with predictable treatments that pose negligible risk."[24]

What's the difference in gingivitis and periodontal disease? Gingivitis is inflammation (redness, swelling and infection) of the gum tissue around teeth. There's no loss of connective tissue and this stage can usually be treated easily. Plaque is usually the cause of gingivitis and periodontal disease. Plaque is the sticky bacteria-infested substance which sticks to teeth. If plaque is not removed, it can harden into a rough deposit on teeth called tartar. If early gingivitis is left untreated, the gums may pull away from the teeth, spaces called "pockets" form and bacteria move in the pockets and begin destroying bone and other support structures of the teeth. As damage progresses, gingivitis becomes periodontal disease, the advanced destructive condition.

Warning signs for gingivitis and periodontal disease include red, swollen, or tender gums which bleed easily when teeth are brushed, gums which have pulled away from teeth, bad breath, loose or separating teeth, pus around teeth or gums, a change in how teeth fit together or how dentures or partial dentures fit. Anyone experiencing these problems should consult a dentist.

Doctors are not saying that gingivitis and periodontal disease cause heart disease. They believe the infection and inflammation of the gums and bone release toxins which affect the endothelial (inside layer) lining of blood vessels, causing the artery walls to become thicker and harder. These thicker, harder artery walls are called atherosclerosis, a part of heart disease. Doctors believe the infection and toxins released in periodontal disease cause other problems for the body. Active infection in the gums and bone can cause infection in other parts of it. Researchers are also finding links between periodontal disease and other serious conditions such as diabetes, kidney disease, and Alzheimer's disease.

Risk factors which increase a person's risk of developing periodontal disease include tobacco smoking or chewing, diabetes, crooked teeth which are hard to clean between, ill-fitting bridges or partial denture sets, and pregnancy. Some medications which contribute to periodontal disease are steroids, cancer therapy drugs, some calcium channel blockers, birth control pills, and some epilepsy drugs.

Can periodontal disease be prevented? The American Dental Association (ADA) recommends: a person should brush his teeth twice a day with fluorie toothpaste and clean between teeth (floss) or use an interdental cleaner once a day.[25] Twice yearly checkups with a dentist will provide plaque/tartar cleaning and a personalized examination including periodic X-rays.

Can periodontal disease be treated? Periodontal disease can often be treated successfully, but it's more complicated and expensive and may require surgical procedures. One procedure called scaling and root planning may also be called deep cleaning or periodontal cleaning by staff at the dental office. This cleaning removes plaque and tartar deposits on teeth and root surfaces. The dentist may need to prescribe antibiotics and pain medications to help clear up the infection and help the person heal the teeth, gums, and bone. For more advanced periodontal disease, surgery may be needed to repair the damage done by the disease.

A person dealing with this situation may wonder if it's worth the time, money and effort. Researchers asked this question: will treatment for periodontal disease improve a person's health? One study reported in the New England Journal of Medicine gave this conclusion: "Intensive periodontal treatment resulted in acute, short-term systemic inflammation and endothelial dysfunction. However, 6 months after therapy, the benefits in oral health were associated with improvement in endothelial function."[26] This study of 120 patients showed that treatment of their severe periodontal disease improved the condition of their blood vessels (inner lining) at six months after the treatment.

Does it matter what toothbrush a person uses? By choosing products with the American Dental Association (ADA) seal of approval, one knows the toothbrush is safe to put in his mouth. The ADA recommends a person buy a toothbrush which fits his mouth so all areas of teeth can be easily cleaned. Both manual and powered toothbrushes can effectively clean teeth provided the person brushes twice a day and cleans all tooth surfaces thoroughly. A dentist may have a recommendation based on the patient's teeth and gums. Powered toothbrushes should be approved by a safety lab such as Underwriters Laboratories (UL). One woman found a powered toothbrush cleaned her teeth better than her manual toothbrush.

Caring for a toothbrush is simple: rinse it after use, store it in an upright position and let it dry. Don't close it in a container, where moist germs would grow easily.

Toothbrushes should be replaced an average of every three to four months. Check your toothbrush and replace it if it's frayed or has worn bristles, as it won't be effective at cleaning the teeth.

Doctors involved in the Austria and Texas research called periodontal disease a risk factor for heart disease. That means a person who has periodontal disease faces an increased risk for developing heart disease. The good news is that gingivitis and periodontal disease for many people are preventable (or treatable if it's already present). These people can eliminate one more risk of heart disease and other conditions to which periodontal disease appears to contribute.

Bad Habits

The *CBS News* headline says it: "Bad habits can age you by 12 years."[27] Four common bad habits — smoking, drinking too much, not exercising and a poor diet — have been linked to aging. During the United Kingdom Health and Lifestyle Survey, researchers looked at 4886 people and their health behaviors. Over a period of 20 years, 1080 of those participants died, 431 from heart/vascular diseases, 318 from cancer and 331 from other diseases. The researchers looked at the four bad habits (smoking, drinking excessive alcohol, not exercising and eating a poor diet) and found that those people with all four bad habits had the same risk of dying as if they had been 12 years older.[28]

During stressful times, a person can take the easy route of fast foods and not exercising. People who enjoy a cigarette may find themselves reaching for one — just to calm the nerves. Caregivers deal with stresses and cares. Only when caregivers make a decision to care for self will they be successful at it.

Section II. Common Health Problems Encountered

11

Alzheimer's Disease

Rring! A pleasant dinner at their favorite restaurant was interrupted for John's family when a phone call grabbed their attention.

"Hello, my name is Susan Jones and I work for Division of Family Services. Is your mother Joan Smith? She wandered away from home and knocked on her neighbor's door. She could not remember your name or phone number. I'm with your mother and you need to come to her house right now." This phone call began the journey into the world of Alzheimer's disease for John's family.

What Is Alzheimer's Disease?

Alzheimer's disease (AD) is a progressive destruction of brain cells, with resulting memory loss. The person affected has increasing difficulty thinking and functioning. While early treatments slow the progression of the disease and make life better for the person and his caregivers, at present Alzheimer's is a fatal brain disease. It is the sixth leading cause of death in America.[1]

Who Develops Alzheimer's Disease and Related Dementias?

No one knows who will develop Alzheimer's or any other dementia. Scientists recognize certain risk factors such as advancing age and genetics.

After age 65, a person's likelihood of developing AD doubles every five years. After age 85, the risk reaches almost 50 percent.[2]

Genetics account for less than 5 percent of Alzheimer's worldwide.[3] This situation is called "familial Alzheimer's disease" and multiple family members in generations within this family are affected. This form of AD occurs early, before age 65, and is caused by gene mutations on chromosomes 1, 14, and 21.[4]

Having a family member (parent, brother, sister, or child) with Alzheimer's disease increases the risk that a person will develop it. Scientists do not know whether this increased risk results from heredity or environmental factors. Could other factors such as a viral or bacterial infection trigger its development?

The majority of Alzheimer's cases are called "late-onset Alzheimer's disease" because a person develops it after age 65. The cause is unknown and as yet, no obvious inheritance pattern has been identified.

Can Alzheimer's Be Prevented or Delayed?

The risk factors of age, family history and genetics cannot be changed. However, scientists believe individuals can influence other risk factors such as head injuries, heart and head health and general healthy aging.

A link between serious head injury and increased risk of AD appears to exist. Individuals can protect their heads by wearing seat belts while in a car, using helmets to prevent sports injuries and preventing falls at home. Fall prevention strategies can be found in chapter 8.

A healthy heart and blood vessel system brings nourishment the human brain needs to function well: "With each heartbeat, arteries carry about 20 to 25% of your blood to your brain, where billions of cells use about 20% of the oxygen and fuel your blood carries. When you are thinking hard, your brain may use up to 50 percent of the fuel and oxygen."[5] Conditions which damage the heart and blood vessels include high blood pressure, heart disease, stroke, diabetes and high cholesterol. Working with their doctors, many individuals can improve their health status and brain health. Healthy aging strategies include controlling one's weight, blood pressure, cholesterol levels and blood sugar levels, exercising, maintaining social connections and avoiding excess alcohol consumption.

Controlling One's Numbers

Keeping body weight, blood sugar, cholesterol and blood pressure numbers within normal limits contributes to good health. The Alzheimer's

Association recommends people practice a healthy life style that includes a low-fat, low-cholesterol diet and exercise. The experts believe lifestyle habits which protect the heart and vascular system of the body promote brain health also.

Doctors Roizen and Oz recommend a healthy diet which promotes cognitive function (thinking, knowing, perceiving). Included in this diet are vitamin-rich colorful vegetables and fruits and healthy omega-3 fishes such as salmon and mahi-mahi: "Among the best nutrients to help keep your cerebral power lines strong are omega-3 fatty acids.... It's been shown that vegetables — any kind, any place — slow cognitive decline even more than fruits. Eating two or more servings a day (just two!) decreases the decline in thinking by 35 percent over six years."[6] The 2009 International Conference on Alzheimer's Disease released information suggesting that a diet which includes grains (complex carbohydrates), low-fat dairy and nuts, green leafy vegetables and oily fish (a Mediterranean type diet) can decrease a person's chances of dementia.[7]

"Type-2 diabetes (the kind associated with being overweight) increases the risk of Alzheimer's, probably by increasing inflammation or arterial aging but also because too much of the hormone insulin in the brain can stimulate beta-amyloid buildup that interferes with the function of cells. In fact, Alzheimer's is now being called type 3 diabetes."[8] While the experts don't know all the details, they believe type 2 diabetes and Alzheimer's disease are connected. Diabetes damages blood vessels and leads to vascular dementia. Diabetics who keep their blood sugar under control through medications or diet and exercise or both protect their vital organs such as heart, kidney and brain.

A condition called prediabetes occurs when a person's body becomes more resistant to the insulin being produced by the person's pancreas. According to Mayo Clinic.Org, a study funded by the National Institute of Diabetes and Digestive and Kidney Diseases found these results: "participants with blood sugar levels slightly above normal (prediabetes) cut their risk of developing type 2 diabetes in half by losing as little as 5 to 7 percent of their body weight and exercising for 30 minutes five days a week. That weight loss translates to 10 to 14 pounds for a 200-pound person."[9] These lifestyle changes will reduce the risk of diabetes, heart attacks, strokes and possibly Alzheimer's disease.

Avoid excess alcohol. The 2009 International Conference on Alzheimer's Disease (ICAD) reported that people with "moderate alcohol intake — those who consume between 8 and 14 drinks per week — are at a 37% lower risk of dementia."[10] Current recommendations say to limit alcoholic beverages to one drink per day for women and two drinks for men.

Exercise. Experts at the 2010 ICAD reported that exercise (walking) can reduce one's risk of developing memory problems: "Scientists at the University of Pittsburgh asked 299 adults, with an average age of 70, how far they walked each week. Nine years later they measured brain size and found people who walked between six and nine miles each week had greater grey matter volume than those walked less. [Their brains had not shrunk.] After 13 years, almost half of the people had developed some form of cognitive impairment." These researchers summarized: "the best way to reduce your risk [of brain shrinkage] is to take regular exercise, eat healthily, don't smoke and get your blood pressure and cholesterol checked."[11]

Social connections matter: "Loneliness is associated with an increased risk of late-life dementia."[12] A group of 823 older persons in Chicago participated in a study looking at loneliness. Over a four-year period, the researchers found that loneliness doubled the risk of developing AD. Emotional isolation or loneliness is bad for brain function.

Does working a crossword or Sudoku puzzle every day protect a person from AD? Doctors followed 488 persons ages 75–85 for five years to see whether cognitive activities affected their memory. Cognitive activity can be defined as conscious, intellectual activity such as thinking, reasoning, and remembering. Their conclusion was that "late life cognitive activities influence cognitive reserve independently of education."[13] In other words, regardless of a person's previous education, doctors found that doing crossword puzzles, reading, writing and other mental activities helps maintain mental function. These mental exercises should be considered a vital part of keeping one's brain healthy.

Symptoms

"Eighty-three percent of us are worried about not being able to remember one another's names. Sixty percent are concerned about our tendency to misplace the car keys. Fifty-seven percent of us are disturbed that we can't recall phone numbers a few minutes after we've heard them.... We are anxious, and our anxiety has a name: Alzheimer's disease."[14] According to the Alzheimer's Association, there are 10 warning signs of Alzheimer's disease.[15]

1. Loss of Memory. Forgetting information recently learned is a common early sign. This forgetting happens more and more often as symptoms

become more obvious. Writing a reminder note becomes useless, as the person cannot use the note for a reminder.
2. Familiar tasks become difficult. A person struggles to perform familiar everyday tasks, such as making a phone call or preparing a meal. For example, Joan's son noticed she cooked less. In times past, Joan could cook an excellent meal but no more.
3. Language problems become apparent. A person forgets familiar words and may substitute unusual words, so his speech doesn't make sense to the listener.
4. Time and place disorientation occurs. The person may become lost in a familiar setting and not know how to return home. Joan would call her son at 2 A.M. just to chat, not realizing it was the middle of the night.
5. Judgment decreases. The person may fall victim to scam artists or may dress inappropriately. Joan agreed to have her house painted by a door-to-door scam artist posing as a painting contractor. When her son learned of this situation, he hurriedly cancelled the job and saved his mother's savings from the scammer.
6. Abstract thinking becomes difficult. A person may struggle with numbers and how to use them. Joan's son noticed his mother's utility bill was overdue and began to ask questions. He saw she was not paying her bills so he began to write out the checks and see that her bills were paid.
7. Objects are misplaced or put in odd places. A person may put car keys in the refrigerator.
8. Mood/personality changes. Joan became very emotional and angry, calling on the telephone and yelling at her son for imagined problems.
9. Trouble understanding visual images and spatial relationships. For some people, vision problems are a sign of Alzheimer's. They may have difficulty judging distance, recognizing color or contrast, even reading. Joan would call the police and her son about intruders in her yard when none could be found.
10. Lack of initiative. A person with Alzheimer's disease may become quiet, sleeping more and not participating in activities around him.

The Alzheimer's Association points out additional information about the differences between normal age-related memory changes and Alzheimer's disease at http://www.alz.org/alzheimers_disease_10_signs_of_alzheimers.asp.

Important Structures and What Happens During Alzheimer's Disease

The human brain weighs three pounds but controls amazing functions. The three major regions of the brain are the cerebrum, cerebellum and brain stem. The cerebrum is the largest part; it controls movement and is involved in functions such as thinking, feeling, solving problems and remembering. The cerebellum can be found at the back of the head and below the cerebrum. The cerebellum controls balance and coordination of the body. The brain stem is located in front of the cerebellum (under the cerebrum) and connects the brain to the spinal cord. Automatic functions of the body such as breathing, blood pressure, heart rate and digestion are controlled by the brain stem.

The brain is fed by arteries bringing blood to it and veins taking used blood away from it. The vascular portion of the brain includes arteries, veins and capillaries. A healthy heart and vascular system means optimal brain function.

The cortex of the brain is the outer wrinkled surface. The different areas of the cortex perform different functions such as thinking, solving problems, remembering, and interpreting the senses such as sight, sounds, and smell. For example, thinking and solving problems occur in the frontal lobe (in the forehead area) while hearing involves the temporal lobe (over the ears).

The 100 billion neurons (nerve cells) of the brain enable human beings to function as humans. These neurons communicate and form networks which enable people to think, learn, and remember. They enable people to use the "senses," to see, hear, smell, etc. By using these nerves, people can move, walking, running and using their muscles in many ways. Alzheimer's disease affects neurons, especially in the hippocampus (the area essential to learning and remembering), the parietal (the area which involves sensation, perception, memory and the senses, especially vision) and the temporal (the area that involves hearing and interpreting what one hears and perceives.[16]

How do the neurons communicate? A thought or memory moves through an individual cell as a tiny electrical charge. When this electrical charge reaches the connection to another cell (a juncture called "synapse"), chemicals known as neurotransmitters are released which carry the signals to the next cell. Alzheimer's disease creates problems for the travel of electrical charges and the neurotransmitter's activities.

Plaques and Tangles

As AD progresses, nerve cells die. These dying cells contain twisted strands of tau protein called "tangles." Instead of normal synapses connecting the cells, abnormal deposits of a protein fragment (beta-amyloid) called "plaques" build up between nerve cells and interfere with normal communication between cells. Scientists believe plaques and tangles interfere with proper function and survival of nerve cells and communication between them.[17] "Alzheimer's disease leads to nerve cell death and tissue loss throughout the brain. Over time, the brain shrinks dramatically, affecting nearly all its functions."[18] An interactive tour of the normal brain and an abnormal Alzheimer's disease brain can be accessed at http://www.alz.org/alzheimers_disease_4719.asp.

Diagnosis

Diagnosis of AD requires the multistep process of a medical workup. There's no one test which can be used to diagnose it. According to the Alzheimer's Association, the steps to a diagnosis include locating the right doctor, who will review the person's health status and medical history and perform a physical examination including a mental and neurological assessment. Diagnostic tests and brain imaging may be performed.

Finding the Right Doctor

Primary care physicians and gerontologists who deal with the elderly may be the first doctor to see their patients and call in specialists to confer. These specialists may include neurologists, who specialize in diseases of the brain and nervous system, psychiatrists, who specialize in the human mind, mood disorders, and mental illnesses and psychologists who test mental functions such as memory, problem solving, language and concentration. Geriatricians are specialists who deal with people aged 50 and older and the medical problems which affect those patients.

Reviewing a Person's Health Status and Medical History

Symptoms of memory loss and confused thinking may be caused in some people by treatable conditions. During the review of medical history and health status, the physicians will look for treatable conditions which could be causing confusion and memory loss such as thyroid problems, kidney or liver disease, diabetes, anemia, malnutrition or certain vitamin deficiencies, excessive use of alcohol, medication side effects, certain infections, and problems with the heart, lung or blood vessels.

A routine check of blood pressure, pulse and temperature will begin the examination. The physician will need an up-to-date list of prescription, herbal supplements and over-the-counter medications the person is taking. The physician will ask questions about diet, nutrition, and the use of alcohol and will also ask about medical conditions for other family members, especially any who have Alzheimer's disease.

Mental Status Test

During the mental status test, the doctor asks a series of questions. He might ask the person to "state the year, season, day of the week and date, and count backward from 100 by 7s or spell 'world' backwards." The doctor would gauge the person's ability to communicate — verbally and through reading and writing — and to care for himself. There are several versions of the mental status tests with a similar goal. The mental exam tells the doctor whether the person is oriented to date and location, how well the person can perform their own care, how well the person can communicate and how well the person can do simple calculations and memory functions.[19]

The physician or specialist will do a neurological examination to assess brain and nervous system function. Parts of the neurological exam include reflexes, eye movements, speech, sensation, coordination and balance, and muscle tone and strength. During this interactive examination, the patient will talk to the doctor, moving as instructed and walking around the exam room. Parts of the exam may feel like a game; for example, the doctor may say, "Hold out your hand, close your eyes and tell me what I place inside your hand." The doctor may place an object such as an ink pen or coin inside the person's hand.[20] This exam gives the physician details of how the brain and nervous system are functioning.

Lab Tests and Brain Imaging Tests

Blood tests and urine tests may be taken to help rule out treatable conditions. For example, a low thyroid level could be causing the patient's symptoms. Brain imaging tests include magnetic resonance imaging (MRI) and computer tomography (CT). These tests give information about the physical size, position and shape of the brain. To look at the function of the brain, positron emission tomography (PET) and functional MRI (fMRI) scans may be done. These two tests indicate how the brain cells use sugar and oxygen.

Dementia Screening Tests for Consumers

The Alzheimer's Association does not recommend the dementia screening tests being developed and marketed to consumers. They believe a home screening test "cannot and should not be used as a substitute for a thorough examination by a skilled doctor.... [A]ny test that plants the idea of a serious illness has the potential to cause great psychological distress to the test taker. The whole process of assessment and diagnosis should be carried out within the context of an ongoing relationship with responsible health care professionals."[21]

Stages of Alzheimer's Disease

According to the Alzheimer's Association, there's a difference between a person's normal aging and Alzheimer's disease. Normal age-related changes include an occasional bad decision, forgetting what day it is but remembering it later, occasionally misplacing items only to find them later, and forgetting to pay a bill or struggling to find a word. By comparison, AD signs include decreasing judgment and ability to make decisions, becoming unable to manage one's budget, losing track of the date or the season, misplacing things and not being able to find them, and experiencing difficulties carrying on a conversation.[22]

The stages of Alzheimer's disease show a progression of symptoms that begins with (in Stage 1) an unimpaired individual with normal function and (in Stage 2) very mild cognitive (perception and knowledge) decline. These may be normal age-related changes or they may decline into Alzheimer's disease. During this stage, the individual may feel he forgets things too much and loses things like glasses or car keys. Other people do not recognize any problems and a medical examination probably would not show any deficit.

Stage 3 brings mild cognitive decline (early Alzheimer's disease). The individual increasingly has difficulties with short-term memory. He can't remember the name of the person he just met. Perhaps he read a magazine article but is unable to remember what he read. He may lose or misplace valuable objects. This individual's decreasing memory and ability to function in work and social settings will become obvious to others such as family, friends and coworkers. During this stage, a medical exam may bring a diagnosis.

Stage 4 is one of moderate cognitive decline (mild or early-stage AD). The individual's decline becomes more obvious to others. This person may seem very withdrawn in social surroundings and cannot remember recent events as well as he did in the past. He has decreased ability to perform complex tasks such as pay bills or planning a meal for company and may not be able to solve challenging math problems as in the past.

Stage 5 is reached when there is moderately severe cognitive decline (moderate or mid-stage Alzheimer's disease). The individual's decline continues. He may have decreased ability to remember details such as current home address and phone numbers but can probably give his name and the names of his immediate family members. He may not be able to remember things from the past such as the name of the college or high school he graduated from. This person may become confused about where he is. He can still usually eat unassisted and manage his bathroom needs. However, choosing proper clothing for the weather may become a problem for this person.

Stage 6 sees severe cognitive decline (moderately severe or mid-stage Alzheimer's disease). The individual's memory and functioning continue to decline. The personality may change and the individual may become suspicious and delusional (believing things which are not true), have hallucinations (seeing or hearing things that aren't there) or begin repetitive behaviors. During this stage, the person may wander and get lost and have sleep disturbances, sleeping during the day and wandering at night. He may no longer recognize loved ones, but generally can distinguish familiar from unfamiliar faces. This person needs increasing help with getting dressed and toileting and may become incontinent of urine and stool.

Stage 7 comes with very severe cognitive decline (severe or late-stage Alzheimer's disease). This final stage of AD finds individuals losing the ability to speak and control their movements. They may need help with eating and all activities of daily living. As the individual declines, he can no longer walk without help or sit without support. Muscles become rigid and swallowing becomes a problem.

Treatments for Alzheimer's Disease

Aricept and Namenda, both familiar names due to television advertising, are approved by the U.S. Food and Drug Administration for treatment of Alzheimer's. Donepezil (Aricept), rivastigmine (Exelon) and galantamine (Razadyne) are cholinesterace inhibitors, which mean they prevent the body from breaking down acetylcholine, one of the chemical messengers involved with memory and learning. These three drugs support nerve cell communication and slow the progression of AD in many people. While rivastigmine and galantamine are used for early to moderate Alzheimer's disease, donepezil (Aricept) is approved for all stages. Memantine (Namenda) works by regulating glutamate, another chemical messenger involved with learning and memory. It's approved for moderate to severe Alzheimer's disease.

Vitamin E may be prescribed to treat AD. An antioxidant, vitamin E may protect nerve cells and delay worsening of symptoms. The Alzheimer's Association recommends "no one should use vitamin E to treat Alzheimer's disease except under the supervision of a physician.... Vitamin E can negatively interact with other medications, including those prescribed to keep blood from clotting."[23]

Doctors may prescribe medications for behavioral and psychiatric symptoms. As the AD progresses, victims may experience delusions, hallucinations, physical and verbal outbursts, and emotional distress. When these symptoms are experienced, the family can try nondrug approaches. Family should recognize the person isn't being mean or difficult but rather is showing disease symptoms. A review by the person's doctor may resolve treatable conditions such as drug side effects. For some, making the home environment feel more comfortable may resolve problems. When nondrug approaches no longer work, drugs may be needed to treat behavior symptoms such as depression or anxiety. Doctors may order antipsychotic drugs to help people suffering from hallucinations, delusions, anger, agitation or hostility. Information on these and all prescription medications can be obtained from the patient's physician, local pharmacists, and the Alzheimer's Association at http://www.alz.org/alzheimers_disease_standard_prescriptions.asp#3.

People wanting information about alternative treatments can access information at the Alzheimer's Association website at http://www.alz.org/alzheimers_disease_alternative_treatments.asp. People with AD often suffer from sleep disorders. Suggested treatments can be accessed at http://www.alz.org/alzheimers_disease_10429.asp.

Research

University of Pennsylvania School of Medicine researchers studying the mouse form of AD are finding that inflammatory cells called microglia contribute to the formation of twisted tau proteins (tangles). These researchers are working to determine whether blocking the inflammatory cells would prevent the tangles and brain damage which results from AD.[24]

Researchers are working to prevent abnormal deposits of beta-amyloid (plaques) in the brain. Phase III clinical trials for the drug Bapineuzumab, an antibody that binds beta-amyloid and helps prevent the accumulation of plaques in the brain, were conducted with the participation of individuals with mild to moderate AD through 2010. Information can be found at http://clinicaltrials.gov/ct2/show/NCT00574132. Researchers around the world are looking at different segments of the Alzheimer's disease process while searching for new treatments and possible vaccine or other preventions. While this science can be confusing to people who sift through all these findings, current important information can be accessed at the Alzheimer's organization Website.

Caregivers and Alzheimer's Disease

Caregivers of those suffering from Alzheimer's disease deal with emotions. It's painful watching a loved one decline from a competent adult to someone who gets lost and wanders away from home. It's heartbreaking when one's beloved wife becomes a frail, forgetful woman who no longer recognizes her husband's face. Caregivers dealing with their many emotions will benefit when they find a good listener, whether a nonjudgmental friend or a professional or a reputable support group. Caregivers need a trusted sounding board to whom they can talk.

Caregivers involved with Alzheimer's disease must recognize the long-term commitment needed and care for themselves. The reality of AD is that it involves years of decline and increasing need for help. Caregivers must be realistic that they must take respite breaks and care for self or they will harm their own health. In her book, *If Only I'd Had This Caregiving Book*, author Maya Hennessey gives a plan caregivers can use to ensure the best care for self and their loved ones. Caregivers can utilize their support network, which can include family, friends, and community resources to provide care to all involved in the caregiving situation.

Also, caregivers must recognize the potential that there will come a time when only one or two people cannot provide the 24/7 care that a person with AD needs. It's not possible. At that time, providing a safe environment and good quality care for the person with AD may require moving the patient to a facility with around-the-clock care and security. Online help with caregiving can be accessed at http://www.alz.org/living_with_alzheimers_caring_for_alzheimers.asp.

The Alzheimer's Research Foundation recommends these practical hints: while helping a person with AD get dressed, limit choices. Because those with AD have difficulty making decisions, offer a choice between "this shirt or this shirt." Another suggestion is to lay out clothing in the order a person will put it on (underwear, socks, pants, shirt, shoes, etc.).[25] Suggestions for mealtime include cutting your own food before you cut up their food (so that person doesn't feel like you're treating them like a baby), and using sauces and gravies to make food more moist and easier to eat. Utensils (knife, fork and spoon) with oversized handles are easier for arthritic hands to use. Fixing breakfast foods for breakfast, lunch foods for lunch and dinner food for dinner will help them stay oriented to time of day.

Traveling with an AD person involves: "bring along an ID tag ... keep things as familiar as possible ... be prepared ... plan your itinerary well in advance ... be realistic ... limit the length of plane or car rides ... if you are driving and the person with Alzheimer's becomes agitated, pull over ... if you are traveling by air, avoid layovers and try to fly on direct flights only ... if you are staying in a hotel, request a large and quiet room ... have a backup plan."[26]

Dr. Michelle Bourgeois, a speech pathology professor, developed a memory book which a caregiving family can use to communicate with their Alzheimer's afflicted loved one. During her research she noticed that people with Alzheimer's could read large-print books and respond appropriately even if they could not retain the words they heard. She designed a book called *My Book of Memories* (which a family can purchase at http://www.northernspeech.com/product/1000012/Cognitive__Linguistic_Disorders/1000090/My_Book_Of_Memories/. The family could make their own memory book by including pictures and printed words large enough that the loved one can read it. These memory books can be used to remind the patient who significant people are and to answer their questions in a way they can retain.[27]

Technology may be helpful to some caregiving families. A baby monitor allows a daughter to hear her mother during the night. When Mom suffers a coughing spell, her daughter can hear and go to Mom's bedroom to check on her. Another technology involves a medical alert system (for example, Lifeline). When Dad fell and could not get himself up off the floor, he pushed the lifeline button around his neck. Utilizing his telephone as a speaker, a Lifeline staff person started calling him by name and asking him if he was ok. This staff person reassured him that help was on the way and called a grandson (listed in their files), who went to Dad's house and picked him up.

A third technology is a home health alert system. Caregiver children can log onto a Website for this alert system and know that their parent's normal routines are occurring that day. Motion sensors can track how often the refrigerator is opened, when a parent gets out of bed and goes to the bathroom, and whether a home health aide arrived for a daily visit. When the normal routines don't occur, the alarm company can notify family to check on their loved one.

People who have Alzheimer's disease will need long-term care. Their caregivers can utilize available resources to care for self while caring for their family member. Until a cure is found for Alzheimer's disease, caregivers must care for self as well as their ill family member.

12

Arthritis

Osteoarthritis (OA) is the most common joint disease, affecting millions around the world. In the United States, OA affects nearly 27 million people. According to the Arthritis Foundation, OA is credited with a total annual cost of $5700 per year for each person living with it.

What Is Arthritis?

Doctors may call it either osteoarthritis or degenerative joint disease (DJD). Osteoarthritis affects the cartilage covering the ends of bones. Normal articular cartilage could be described as translucent, white and smooth. At the end of a chicken leg, the smooth shiny covering visible is articular cartilage. This cartilage enables bones to glide smoothly and painlessly.

When degenerative changes to the cartilage occur, it becomes a dull white and develops hair-like projections called fibrillations. The joint may become deformed and bone spurs develop. If these bone spurs, called "osteophytes," break off, they float around inside the joint, causing pain and possibly more damage. When the cartilage wears off the ends of a bone, a person may be walking on "bone-on-bone." This person probably experiences pain, stiffness, grating or catching sensations within the joint. As the cartilage failed, osteoarthritis or degenerative joint disease occurred.

Osteoarthritis affects only joints, unlike some other types of arthritis, such as rheumatoid arthritis, which involves the whole body. The joints most often affected by OA include the fingers and hands, the neck (cervical) and lower spine (lumbar area) and weight bearing joints of knees and hips.

Who Gets Arthritis?

Men experience OA more than women until age 50. After age 50, women are more often affected than men. For many people symptoms of osteoarthritis begin after age 40. Younger people can develop OA as a result of an injury to joints, a congenital (present at birth) joint problem or an inherited defect in the cartilage. Causes of osteoarthritis include heredity, injury — whether from sports or job-related or any other cause — overuse, and lifestyle behaviors such as inactivity and being overweight.

Scientists recognize a genetic basis for the development of osteoarthritis. One gene mutation which makes cartilage more fragile has been identified. The genetic factor involving OA of the hands may be as high as 65 percent.[1] Researchers recognize that the daughters of women who have knee arthritis deal with knee arthritis also. However, "genetics alone cannot explain all the development of osteoarthritis because identical twins do not experience osteoarthritis in the huge percentages expected."[2]

Injuries can contribute to osteoarthritis. "Major acute knee injuries, including cruciate ligament and meniscal tears, are common causes of knee OA."[3] The anterior and posterior cruciate ligaments are stabilizing structures inside the knee which prevent excess motion. The menisci (both medial and lateral) are cushions which protect the knee joint from injuries. Sports activities which can contribute to injuries and development of osteoarthritis include marathon running (hip OA), soccer (both knee and hip OA) and football (knee OA). Job injuries can increase a person's risk of OA. For example, farmers have increased risk of hip OA, while jackhammer operators have increased risk of developing osteoarthritis in their elbows.

According to the Arthritis Foundation, lifestyle behaviors such as lack of exercise and being overweight can contribute to development of OA: "Weight control is important for prevention of and to slow the progression of OA affecting the weight-bearing joints (knees and hips) and low back."[4] Even a small weight loss can decrease the risk of developing knee osteoarthritis: "For every pound of weight loss, there is a four pound reduction in the load exerted on the knee for each step taken during daily activities."[5] Exercise recommendations include those programs that are easy on joints. Low-impact exercises such as walking, tai chi for arthritis, and aquatic activities can keep a person's joints flexible and fit.

Symptoms

Pain sends people to their doctors. This pain may affect only one joint or multiple joints. It may begin gradually and increase over time. A person may find he has pain and stiffness in those joints after excessive use or after times of rest. A grating and catching sensation may occur. Bony growths called osteophytes or bone spurs may appear on X-rays. Osteoarthritis symptoms may also include swelling and tenderness in joints.

"Gel phenomenon" refers to the stiffness a person may experience after periods of inactivity. This stiffness resolves within minutes when the person begins to walk and move.

Important Structures and What Happens

Articular cartilage covers the end of bones and acts as a shock absorber and friction reducer. This cartilage is made of 65 percent to 80 percent water, chondrocytes and proteins called collagen and proteoglycans. Chondrocytes are cells (cytes) which build cartilage (chondro). Collagen is a colorless, fibrous protein that the body uses when building skin, bone and connective tissue. Proteoglycan is a sugar-protein substance which gives cartilage the ability to resist compression. Collagen and proteoglycan are woven together into the structure of articular cartilage. Healthy cartilage provides smooth movement free of pain.

The human skeleton is made up of 206 bones. A person may be surprised to learn that bones are living tissue with an internal blood supply. The human body has a constant cycle of breaking down old bone and building new bone. Articular cartilage is no different. A normal cycle occurs where the articular cartilage is broken down and rebuilding occurs. Osteoarthritis occurs when there's a "failure of chondrocytes (cartilage cells) within the joint to synthesize a good-quality matrix [articular cartilage], in terms of resistance and elasticity, and to maintain the balance between synthesis and degradation of the extracellular matrix."[6] "After osteoarthritis begins, the ability of chondrocytes to make good quality cartilage decreases while these cells produce increased enzymes to break down the cartilage."[7] As the cartilage becomes soft, it's more fragile and prone to injury. Doctors call this chondromalacia [softening of cartilage]. Damage continues as the cartilage wears thin and holes develop, exposing raw bone.

Scientists continue to look for answers to what causes osteoarthritis: Do enzymes called cytokines contribute to increased breakdown that the body cannot repair quickly enough? Why do chondrocytes fail to build new cartilage as quickly as it's needed?

Diagnosis

A trip to the doctor can bring a diagnosis of osteoarthritis. The doctor will begin with a history and physical and will ask questions about the pain, stiffness and function of the joint(s) and how the symptoms are affecting the person's lifestyle and daily activities. The doctor will want a list of all medications, including over-the-counter and herbal drugs. A physical examination will be needed. For pain in the spine, knee, or hip, the doctor may ask the person to walk and show him where the pain is occurring and other pertinent details.

X-rays may be ordered. While early arthritis may not show up on X-rays, more advanced cases will show changes: joint space narrowing, subchondral bony changes and osteophytes (bone spurs).[8] In some cases, an magnetic resonance imaging (MRI) X-ray will be ordered. Lab work may be drawn to rule out other possibilities such as rheumatoid arthritis. Because osteoarthritis isn't a systemic disease (affecting the entire body), lab work is usually within normal limits. A joint aspiration may be recommended. During the joint aspiration, fluid from inside the joint is drained using a syringe and needle. This fluid is sent to a lab for examination and ruling out other forms of arthritis.

Finding the Right Doctor

A family doctor, or primary care doctor, is an excellent and needed resource. This doctor can provide the needed history, physical exam, tests and X-rays to diagnose and treat osteoarthritis and may send the patient to a specialist if needed. A rheumatologist is a doctor who uses medical treatments for arthritis and related conditions. An orthopaedic surgeon specializes in surgical procedures to treat bone and joint diseases. For example, many orthopaedic surgeons perform total joint replacement surgeries.

Physical therapists and occupational therapists are both excellent resources that a person dealing with arthritis may need. Physical therapists teach people how to improve their joint function using exercises which will strengthen and improve a person's strength and agility. They teach a person how to use crutches or a walker the person will need while recuperating from surgery. Occupational therapists teach a person how to perform activities of daily living with a minimum of pain, including people recovering from hip surgery, who must dress themselves in such a way as to minimize the risk of dislocating their hip.

Other resources may include social workers who help a person dealing with financial and job-related difficulties due to physical conditions.

Emotion and Mental Aspects of Arthritis

Pain is depressing to the person dealing with it. "Depression, anxiety and feelings of helplessness" can interfere with daily life for a person and his family.[9] Osteoarthritis can also impact a person's finances because of the cost of treatment and wages lost due to OA and its resulting disabilities.

The Arthritis Foundation recommends a person visit his doctor for recommendations, learn about osteoarthritis and take charge of his life. The "Self-Help Course" offered through chapters of the Arthritis Foundation teaches a person how to better manage pain, exercise safely, manage fatigue and stress, better communicate with his doctor, and other valuable tools. The *Arthritis Helpbook* also provides self-management tactics which enable a person to take charge of his life and improve coping skills.

Treatments

The goals for OA treatment involve controlling pain and improving joint function while maintaining normal body weight and achieving a healthy lifestyle.[10] The experts at the Arthritis Foundation recommend multiple strategies for pain management. These strategies include exercise, pain medicines, complementary and alternative therapies such as massage and acupuncture, and nondrug treatments such as heat and cold treatments and surgery.

"Physical fitness for people is much like good maintenance and proper use for an automobile. Both allow you to start when you want, enjoy a smooth and relaxed trip, get to your destination without a breakdown, and have some fuel in your tank when you arrive. How well an automobile works depends on its points and plugs, filters, hoses, tires, lubrication and fuel systems. Your physical fitness is important in determining how easy and comfortable it is for you to do what you want and need to do every day."[11]

Most people will find that when they exercise, they experience an improved mood, decreased amount of pain and more flexibility in their joints. Before beginning exercises, a person should talk with his doctor about what exercises he should do. Three types of exercise are recommended. Aerobic exercises get a person's heart pumping and keep his lungs and circulatory system healthy. As a person does aerobic exercise such as walking or swimming, his stamina increases and his heart becomes stronger. Gentle-to-joint aerobic exercises include walking, swimming, or low-impact aerobics such as tai chi for arthritis and water aerobics. Strengthening exercises involve light weights or elastic bands. A person using these weights or bands will strengthen the muscles of his body and protect his joints.

Range-of-motion exercises help keep joints flexible and able to move. A person does range-of-motion exercises by slowly and easily turning the head to the right, then to the left. Next he should tilt his head toward one shoulder and then toward the other, exhaling when the head moves down and inhaling when the head comes up. Range of motion exercises should always be gentle and at a slow pace without bouncing. All exercises should be approved by one's doctor or physical therapist as being gentle to joints; exercises should not cause severe pain. A person beginning a new exercise program should begin by using little weights and few repetitions and gradually increase them.

Pain medications commonly used for osteoarthritis include analgesics and nonsteroidal anti-inflammatory drugs (NSAIDS). Analgesics are pain pills such as acetaminophen (Tylenol) which relieve pain but do nothing for inflammation. Acetaminophen, an inexpensive over-the-counter drug, is considered a first choice drug for osteoarthritis pain. For severe pain, doctors may prescribe an analgesic with narcotic (opioid).

Aspirin, the first nonsteroidal anti-inflammatory drug (NSAID), was marketed in 1899 by the Friedrich Bayer & Co. NSAIDs help control pain, decrease inflammation in joints, decrease fever and prolong blood clotting by affecting platelet function. The drugs all block prostaglandins (hormone-like substances in the body which contribute to inflammation and pain). NSAIDs are divided into three categories: traditional NSAIDS, COX-2 inhibitors and salicylates.

Traditional NSAIDs include 20 different medications. Some NSAIDS are available over the counter, such as ibuprofen (Advil or Motrin) and naproxen (Aleve). All traditional NSAIDS can have side effects of stomach upset and bleeding of the gastrointestinal (GI) tract. Researchers working to decrease the GI side effects developed COX-2 inhibitors (a newer version of NSAIDs). When refecoxib (Vioxx) first came out in 1999, it seemed a wonder drug for people dealing with arthritis pain because it relieved their pain and caused less GI upset. Over the next five years, over 91 million prescriptions were written in the U.S. The wonder drug came under scrutiny when a scientific study asked whether refecoxib could prevent colon polyps. This study found a significant risk of heart attack and strokes among study participants and refecoxib was pulled off the market.

Since that time researchers have realized all NSAIDs carry significant risks. Doctors are recognizing that senior citizens face increased risks of heart attack and stroke when they take any NSAID. Each individual should talk with his doctor about his pain level and the best, safest way to manage his pain. Caregivers of those people should talk to the person's doctor before using NSAIDS, including any over-the-counter type.

The third type of NSAID, salicylates, include aspirin and a chemical variation called nonacetylated salicylate, which should have fewer side effects. Nonacetylated salicylate doesn't have the heart protective side effect that aspirin possesses.

Two treatments for osteoarthritis will be done in the doctor's office or clinic setting: Corticosteroid injection and Viscosupplement injections. Corticosteroid injections are commonly called "steroid shots" or "cortisone shots." A cortisone shot involves the doctor injecting a small amount of the steroid into the painful joint. The medication decreases the inflammation and pain the person feels in that joint. The physician judges the success of the cortisone shot by the decreased symptoms the patient experiences. If a person only gets a few days of relief, the cortisone shot isn't considered a success. Doctors limit the number of steroid shots because of possible side effects.

Viscosupplement (hyaluronic acid) injections replace hyaluronic acid. Hyaluronic acid, a shock absorber and lubricant in joint fluid, is deficient in people who have osteoarthritis. In theory, replacing the hyaluronic acid will improve the function of the joint while decreasing pain and inflammation. The hyaluronic acid injections will be a series of weekly injections of either three or five, depending on the product. Two hyaluronic acid products are Hyalgan and Synvisc. Hyaluronic acid seems to have anti-inflammatory and pain-relieving benefits which may last for several months. "The injections may also stimulate the body to produce more of its own hyaluronic acid."[12]

Another option in pain medications is the use of topical analgesics (creams, rubs or salves) applied directly to the painful area. Voltaren Gel, a topical version of diclofenac, an NSAID, is available by prescription. Other topicals include the over-the-counter products of capsaicin, counterirritants and salicylates. Patients should discuss the use of topical analgesics with their doctor and follow instructions for safe usage.

Capsaicin (an ingredient found in cayenne peppers) works by stimulating and overpowering the neurotransmitter which sends pain messages to the brain. The person may notice stinging, burning or itching when it's applied in the first couple weeks of use, but this stinging, burning or itching should decrease. Some product names for capsaicin are Zostrix, Zostrix HP, and Capzasin-P.

Counterirritants work when they distract a person's brain from the pain by using a sensation of heat or cold to irritate nerve endings. Menthol, oil of wintergreen, camphor and eucalyptus are some of the substances used in counterirritants. Commonly used counterirritant products include ArthriCare, Eucalyptamint, Icy Hot and Therapeutic Mineral Oil. Salicylates can be found in topical form such as Aspercreme, Ben-Gay, Flexall and Sportscreme. These topical products work as counterirritants but may also inhibit prostaglandins.

All topical analgesic products should be used as directed by the manufacturers. Safety instructions for capsaicin, counterirritants and topical salicylates are similar. These topical medications are for external use. A word of warning: patients should wash their hands thoroughly after using capsaicin and avoid touching eyes or moist mucous membranes (such as nose, throat, lips, urethra, vagina or rectum) with the capsaicin product on his hands. Avoid getting these topical medications on unhealed areas of skin. Do not use a heating pad or tightly bandage an area of the body while any of these medications are on it. A person should consult his doctor if severe skin irritation, redness, swelling or an increase in the joint pain occurs during use of capsaicin products. These products should not be used on children under 12 years of age unless a doctor directs the usage. These products should be kept safely away from children and if accidentally ingested, a doctor or poison center should be contacted immediately. If symptoms of allergic reaction occurs (itching, swelling of the face, wheezing, a feeling of apprehension or anxiety, difficulty breathing or swallowing), call 911 for emergency assistance.

Alternative and Complementary Medicine

The 2007 survey of over 23,000 Americans (age 18 and above) found that 38 percent of adults and 12 percent of children use complementary and alternative medicine (CAM). A few CAM treatments considered beneficial to osteoarthritis sufferers include acupuncture, biofeedback, massage, meditation, prayer, relaxation, tai chi, and yoga.

People wanting information about which CAM treatments are considered safe and effective for osteoarthritis can find Arthritis Foundation books, such as *Alternative Treatments for Arthritis* by Dorothy Foltz-Gray, to be valuable resources.

Acupuncture

Acupuncture relieves pain and improves function in knee osteoarthritis. A National Institutes of Health 2004 news report lends support to the use of acupuncture for knee osteoarthritis pain and function. Researchers worked with 570 people aged 50 and older who had osteoarthritis of the knee. The three choices in the research were acupuncture, simulated acupuncture and a control group who followed the Arthritis Foundation's self-help program. This research followed these participants for 26 weeks: "Overall, participants in the acupuncture group had a 40 percent decrease in pain and a nearly 40 percent improvement in function compared to their assessments at the start of the study."[13]

Acupuncture practices began in ancient Chinese medicine. This philosophy believes a vital force of energy called qi (pronounced chee) flows through the body in invisible channels called meridians. When the energy (qi) flows freely through all the meridians, good health is present. When a blockage of the energy occurs, disease, dysfunction or pain occurs. "Very fine needles inserted into the skin along the meridians can correct the flow of qi, restoring balance and blocking pain."[14] Western scientists speculate that acupuncture works by stimulating the central nervous system to release endorphins and other pain-blocking chemicals.

When looking for an acupuncturist, a person should begin by asking his doctor for a referral. Medical doctors who practice acupuncture can be found at The American Academy of Medical Acupuncture Website at http://www.medicalacupuncture.org/. Certified acupuncture practitioners can be found at the National Certification Commission for Acupuncture and Oriental Medicine at http://www.nccaom.org/ or the American Association of Oriental Medicine at http://www.aaaomonline.org/.

"Acupuncture is considered safe if it is done by a licensed practitioner with sterilized, disposable needles."[15] Before any treatment, the acupuncturist should ask about medical history including all medications — prescription, herbal and over-the-counter. During the medical history, a person should tell the acupuncturist about the presence of breast implants or a pacemaker as well as a current pregnancy. The acupuncturist should prevent infection by cleansing the area of skin with alcohol and using sterile, disposable needles.

Biofeedback

"Biofeedback uses modern-day technology to monitor certain body functions and enable a person to learn control over those functions. By wearing sensors, a person can either see squiggly lines or hear beeps that indicate body functions such as pulse, body temperature, muscle tension, or digestion. The person can learn to control the beeps or squiggles through relaxation techniques."[16] Some bodily functions that a person can control using biofeedback include blood pressure, brain activity, heart rate, muscle tension, bowel and bladder problems, and digestion.

A person who wants to learn biofeedback should consult his doctor, especially if he has a pacemaker, heart problems or diabetes. Biofeedback techniques are learned through a series of lessons on techniques that have been approved by the National Institutes of Health for treatment of insomnia and pain.

Massage Therapy

Massage is an ancient practice from the Indian Ayurvedic beliefs. A survey taken in 2009 showed almost a third of Americans (32 percent) get massages for health and medical reasons. Increasing numbers of people recognize that massage therapy can help reduce pain (86 percent) while 85 percent agree that massage contributes to a person's good health.[17] Massage is used to relax muscles, decrease pain and relieve stress and tension. More than 100 types of massage are performed. Some common forms include Swedish massage, deep tissue massage, trigger point therapy and reflexology.

A person's doctor can refer him to a massage therapist. Online sources include the National Certification Board for Therapeutic Massage and Body at www.ncbtmb.com or the American Massage Therapy Association at www.amtamassage.org. Candidates for massage should discuss massage therapy with their doctor, as some types of massage can "worsen high blood pressure, osteoporosis or circulatory problems."[18] Women should tell the massage therapist if they're pregnant. Tell the therapist to avoid areas where skin is damaged, open, or painful.

Meditation

Meditation begins when a person finds a quiet place, begins taking several big deep breaths, and quiets his mind. He can focus on a word, a sound, a thought or a sensation. As this person relaxes, he should find peacefulness. During this meditation time, a person's stress and pain can fade away, leaving him refreshed and calm.

Meditation, another ancient practice, has been a part of both Eastern and Western religious practices for centuries. In Western countries, many people mix it with prayer. The goal of meditation is to reach a state of "thoughtless awareness, during which a person is passively aware of sensations at the present moment."[19] Studies have shown that one practicing meditation can lower his blood pressure, slow his heart rate and decrease the level of stress hormones in his body.[20]

Persons wanting to learn meditation should take a class with an experienced instructor. Meditation can raise powerful, unresolved emotions and actually increase anxiety for some individuals. An experienced instructor can be helpful.

Prayer

Prayer and religious practices can be added to meditation as a part of CAM practices. For many people, prayer is an integral part of life. They pray for their own health (43 percent). They ask others to pray for their health (24 percent) and 10 percent of Americans participate in a prayer group for their own health.[21] A 2006 Gallup poll found that 73 percent of Americans believe God exists (believe it as a certainty).[22]

A 2010 Gallup poll found that very religious people lead healthier lives. "Very religious" is defined in this study: "religion is an important part of daily life and church/synagogue/mosque attendance occurs at least every week or almost every week." A total of 43.7 percent of Americans fit in this category. This poll found the very religious smoke less, get regular exercise and eat healthier food when compared to moderately religious and nonreligious Americans.[23]

Visualization

Visualization can be added to meditation when a person focuses on a mental picture. A person could close his eyes, relax and become mentally transported to a Caribbean beach. As he breathes deeply, he can visualize: seeing turquoise blue waters and feeling a warm breeze on his pain-free body.

Tai Chi

Tai chi combines meditation and slow fluid movements. This Chinese martial art practice combines mental focus, deep breathing and slow movements to balance the life energy called qi. The gentle movements of tai chi have made it an exercise that people with arthritis can use to improve muscle strength and decrease their pain levels. Multiple studies have shown that tai chi adapted for arthritis is a successful treatment. Another benefit of tai chi is improved balance and muscle strength, which prevented falls in study participants.

Yoga

Yoga, another ancient Indian Ayurveda healing practice, uses emphasis on the mental, physical and spiritual aspects. The word "yoga" means union and its practice bring a person's body, mind and spirit into harmony. Several types of yoga are practiced around the world. One type called bhakti yoga focuses on spirituality. The hatha type of yoga is commonly practiced in the U.S. Yoga enthusiasts find that the gentle stretches, meditation and slow deep breathing yield results of lower blood pressure and stress and they experience increased muscle tone, flexibility, balance and energy.

A person who wants to learn yoga should ask his doctor if there are any yoga poses he should avoid and be sure to talk to the yoga instructor about any physical limitations he might have before starting class.

Heat Treatments

A warm bath can ease arthritis pain by increasing blood flow while decreasing the inflammation and relaxing tight muscles in the affected areas. Other ways to utilize heat is to apply an electric heating pad or a heat wrap made for the painful area of body. A word of caution about the electric heating pad: over 100,000 people burn themselves every year when they fall asleep with the heating pad turned on or when they use topical analgesic creams with the heating pad. Avoid this danger.[24]

Surgery performed for arthritis includes total joint replacement. Chapter 7 gives information about preoperative, during surgery and postoperative care of a person having surgery.

Prevention

Can osteoarthritis be prevented? What do the experts say? No one knows whether a person can prevent osteoarthritis. However, the Arthritis Foundation recommendations state that healthy living habits play a role in preventing OA. Suggestions include eating a healthy diet, maintaining a recommended body weight, using good posture, exercising regularly with gentle-to-joints activities, avoiding smoking and limiting alcohol intake. They suggest a person talk to his doctor about vitamin and mineral supplements and preventing osteoporosis for bone health.

Many children and young adults become involved in sports activities. Using proper equipment can protect them from injuries. The American Academy of Orthopaedic Surgeons provides safety information and prevention strategies at http://orthoinfo.aaos.org/menus/safety.cfm.

Can a person's shoes contribute to osteoarthritis? Dr. Casey Kerrigan's work says yes, as her research shows that women's high heel shoes can contribute to knee osteoarthritis. Dr. Kerrigan began by studying stiletto heels (2.75 inches), which she found increased the pressure on knee joints by 22 percent. When Dr. Kerrigan studied wider heels versus narrow heels, she found wider heels contributed at least the same force on the knee joint as narrow heels. Over the years she has studied lower heels and found that the lower the heels of the shoe, the less pressure there is on knee joints. Dr. Kerrigan is quoted as saying this: "Heels are bad, whether they are thin or wide. My recommendation is simple and unpopular — it's to wear no heels at all."[25]

Research

Researchers have recognized for many years that overweight and obese people have increased risk of developing OA, especially in weight bearing joints like knees. New research points to an explanation. They're recognizing that "fat" secretes cytokines (signaling molecules) and may contribute to osteoarthritis not only in knees but also in the wrist and hands.[26]

What do the researchers say about glucosamine and chondroitin supplements? The first Glucosamine/Chondroitin Arthritis Intervention Trial (GAIT) was undertaken to determine whether glucosamine and chondroitin supplements were an effective treatment for OA pain in the knee. The participants of this study were divided into five groups taking medication: (1) glucosamine alone, (2) chondroitin sulfate alone, (3) glucosamine and chondroitin sulfate in combination, (4) celecoxib (Celebrex) or (5) a placebo (an inactive substance that looks like the study pill). After six months of participation, the results of this study found that the patients taking celecoxib experienced significant pain relief. Overall, the glucosamine, chondroitin and combination of glucosamine and chondroitin treated osteoarthritis pain equal to a placebo for people with mild pain. A small group of participants with moderate-to-severe pain did receive significant pain relief from the glucosamine/chondroitin combination. This study was reported in 2006.

Stage 2 of the GAIT study involved participants who continued for an additional 18 months. Stage 2 was held to determine whether glucosamine/chondroitin supplements prevent osteoarthritic joint damage. The results were based on X-ray comparisons of study participants. After two years (six months of the first GAIT study plus eighteen months of the second GAIT study) the X-ray results found none of the treatments showed significant prevention of osteoarthritis damage.[27] Ongoing research being sponsored by the Arthritis Foundation can be found at http://www.arthritis.org/research-update.php. Ongoing research about arthritis that is being sponsored by the National Center for Complementary and Alternative Medicine can be found at http://nccam.nih.gov/research/results/spotlight/atoz.htm.

Caregivers and the Disease

Caregivers find themselves dealing with osteoarthritis in their loved one and may find they have osteoarthritis pain in their own body. The recommendations from experts at the Arthritis Foundation, the National Institutes of Health and the American Academy of Orthopaedic Surgeons can help guide caregivers in dealing with this all too common disease.

13

Cancer

Driving his car down the highway, C. Kip Bennett felt that he had peanut butter stuck to the roof of his mouth. Strange, he thought to himself as he flipped down the visor, glanced in the mirror, and saw something white in the back of his throat. Since it was a Thursday afternoon, he stopped at a local medical clinic. The doctor recommended antibiotics and a return visit for the next week. On the return visit to the clinic, the doctor said, "We've got to send you someplace fast. It's not what I thought it was. It's growing fast and has a necrotic [dead tissue] center." Anxiety became Kip's constant companion.

The next few weeks involved multiple doctor visits, tests such as a chest X-ray, CT scan, and a biopsy of the white mass in the back of Kip's throat. Worry and fear ran through his mind as he heard an ear, nose and throat (ENT) surgeon give the diagnosis of Stage 3 (almost stage 4) squamous cell carcinoma of Kip's tonsils. The doctor told Kip at stage 4 there's little chance of beating the cancer. Kip's cancer was growing so fast it was outgrowing its blood supply and it had invaded five lymph nodes in Kip's body.

Kip had to make decisions about treatment. Should he have a radical neck dissection surgery as recommended by one ENT surgeon? The surgeon told him that radical neck surgery would involve the surgeon breaking his jaw and removing large amounts of tissue from his neck and throat. Would it be necessary to remove his larynx (voice box) leaving him unable to speak? Should he get a second opinion? Should he travel to one of the world's premier cancer hospitals? The doctors were saying the cancer was growing fast. What should he do? Because the local hospital was affiliated with a Houston, Texas, premier cancer hospital, an appointment was made there and within ten days Kip found himself traveling to Texas to get a second opinion.

Kip's cancer was rare. "If I've got the statistics right, in 2007 there were 7000 cases of tonsillar cancer in the world. If you go to someone who has treated 3000 of those 7000 cases your chance of coming out with a good result are so much better. I would say find the right doctor for your type of cancer" is Kip's advice.[1]

At the Houston cancer hospital, Kip met with a team comprising a radiologist, an oncologist and an ENT surgeon who gathered pertinent information about his health status and made a recommendation: 47 radiation treatments with 3 weeks of chemotherapy. They told Kip, "We're pretty sure we can get this cancer. We feel safe in telling you, if there's any levity in the situation, the only way you're going to die in Houston is if you get hit by a bus on the way to an appointment." Kip remembers, "that made me laugh and at that point I wasn't doing much laughing."[2]

Cancer — What Is It?

Cancer could be called "cells gone bad" or uncontrolled cell growth. Normally cells grow and stop growing in a programmed fashion. When the cell growth goes awry and the new cells are different from the old cells, these abnormal cells may continue to grow abnormally and past the point where their growth should have stopped. The new abnormal growth is called "neoplasm," or new growth.

Neoplasm can refer to benign or malignant growths. A benign neoplasm is not cancer. A benign neoplasm is a growth that will continue to expand at a slow rate and at the location where it originated. It usually has a fibrous tissue covering over it and rarely causes death unless its expanding size puts pressure on vital functions of the body.

A malignant neoplasm is cancer. Cancer grows and can invade surrounding tissues, as well as break off cells which travel to distant parts of the body, reattach, and cause metastases (meaning cancer cells have spread to other areas of the body). The cancer cells which metastasize do so via the blood or lymphatic systems.

The Demographics of Who Gets Cancer

In 2007, a total of 1.45 million Americans were diagnosed with cancer and more than 559,000 of them died with cancer that same year.[3] The

American Cancer Society (ACS) expects a slightly larger number (1.529 million) diagnosed in 2010. In 2006, over 2 million cases of skin cancer — basal, squamous and melanoma — were treated.[4]

Cancer involves over 100 different and distinctive diseases. For men, prostate cancer continues to be the largest number of newly diagnosed cases (28 percent). For women, breast cancer accounts for the most newly diagnosed cases of cancer (28 percent). However, the leading cause of death from cancer for both men and women is lung cancer. While heart disease is the number one killer of Americans, lung cancer ranks second as a cause of death.

Five-year survival rates (for years 1999 to 2005) for all cancers have increased to 68 percent due to earlier diagnosis and improved treatments. This rate refers to the percentage of cancer patients who are alive at the five-year mark when compared to those not having cancer.

Symptoms

The experts at the American Cancer Society recommend that a person see a doctor if he develops any of the following symptoms: a change in bowel habits or bladder function, sores that don't heal, any unusual bleeding or discharge, thickening or lump in the breast or other areas of the body, a nagging cough or hoarseness, recent changes in a mole or any new skin change, indigestion or difficulty swallowing, and white patches inside the mouth or on the tongue. Nonspecific symptoms include unexplained weight loss (as much as or more than 10 lbs.), fever, fatigue, pain and skin changes.[5]

Important Structures of the Body and What Happens

"There are more than 300 trillion cells in the human body and every second of every day more than 10 million die and are replaced."[6] Some cells such as bone marrow cells and lymphocytes (a type of white blood cells which helps protect a person's immune status) have a short life and must replicate often. Other cells such as liver cells seldom replicate themselves. Scientists believe the liver cells replicate themselves about once a year unless an injury or illness occurs and the liver needs to repair itself.[7]

When scientists talk about cells, they use words like nucleus (the control center of the cell), mitochondria (the powerhouse of the cell) and deoxyribonucleic acid (DNA, or the genetic material of cells). The inner workings of cells are an amazingly complex group of activities. A normal cell cycle involves a series of steps that result in a person's genetic information being duplicated exactly into a new cell; the body's old cell then dies when its replacement is ready.

The concern about cancer is in regard to this cell reproduction. When a disorder occurs during cell reproduction, a neoplasm occurs. Doctors have noted that the neoplasm (new abnormal cells) grows uncontrolled; it grows and increases in size, crowding and interfering with normal cell growth and function. When cancer occurs, the cells do not heed the body's normal shut-down mechanisms, so old cells don't die; the new cancer cells continue to grow haphazardly and uncontrolled.

Diagnosis/Lab Tests/Imaging Tests/ Screening Tests

Screening for some types of cancer is well known. Mammograms, colonoscopy, and Pap smear tests are recommended on a regular basis. Cancer is easier to cure when it's found early. Every person should discuss his risk of developing cancer with his doctor and follow the doctor's recommendation for screening tests.

General recommendations from the American Cancer Society (ACS) include yearly mammograms for women age 40 and above and some type of colon cancer test after age 50 for both men and women. The colon cancer test may be an X-ray procedure such as barium enema every 5 years or an endoscopy procedure such as flexible sigmoidoscopy every 5 years or colonoscopy every 10 years. To detect cervical cancer, a Pap smear test should be performed on a regular basis as recommended by a woman's doctor.

Blood tests to find cancer are called tumor markers. One blood test being used for this purpose is the prostate-antigen test (PSA). Because of inaccuracies in this test — positive results due to noncancerous prostate conditions or negative (normal) results in some men who have prostate cancer — the American Cancer Society recommends that each man discuss with his doctor whether to have a PSA test at age 50 (age 45 for African American men and men whose father, son or brother has had a history of prostate cancer).[8]

There are a variety of radiological tests used to detect cancers and to determine the effectiveness of treatments for people undergoing cancer treatments. Some of these radiology tests include X-rays, CT scans, MRI scans, mammograms and nuclear medicine scans such as bone scans and PET (positive emission tomography) scans. These tests give doctors information without surgical intervention.

An X-ray (also called radiograph) produces black, gray and white images. It's a readily available and inexpensive technology which produces an image that can be used to detect some tumors. For example, a chest X-ray will show diseases affecting the lungs, including cancer. Sometimes X-ray dye (contrast) is injected to increase the information doctors can gain from the X-ray.

A CT scan (also called CAT scan) is a computer tomography scan. CT scans can show a tumor's size and shape, its location, and whether it has blood vessels attached to it. These scans show a cross-section slice of the body. Doctors gain valuable information about the success of cancer treatments when they compare CT scans done at different time periods, maybe months or years apart. A CT scan can be done without X-ray dye or with X-ray dye. If dye is used, it can be swallowed, injected into a vein or inserted as an enema. Dye gives the CT scan contrast because different tissues absorb dye differently.

MRI (magnetic resonance imaging) X-rays also produce cross-section views of the body, but they are accomplished through a technology using magnets inside the machine. MRIs may be used to detect cancer in the brain and head, spine, bones and muscles.

Mammogram is an X-ray of breast tissue. It's used as a screening tool to identify early breast cancer.

Nuclear medicine X-rays include several tests, such as bone scans and PET scans. Nuclear scans use the body's chemistry to make pictures. A special radioactive substance called a tracer or radionuclide is injected into a person's body and the machine records the absorption of the tracer into specific body tissues. These scans find tumors in multiple parts of the body such as bones, lungs, and thyroid. They can be used to determine how well cancer treatment is working. Bone scans help doctors identify bone cancers.

PET (positive emission tomography) scans utilize a radioactive sugar which is absorbed at different rates by cells, depending on how fast those cells are growing. Because cancer cells grow fast, they absorb the radioactive sugar in larger amounts. The PET scan is used for studying the brain and finding many cancers, including head and neck, thyroid, colon, breast, lung, ovary, melanoma and lymphoma.

Combining a PET scan and CT scan has resulted in a machine which helps doctors locate areas of increased cellular activity, which often indicates the site of tumors. Researchers continue developing new technologies which help in the screening and diagnosis of cancers.

Finding the Right Doctor

A family practice doctor, primary care physician, or nurse practitioner may be the first doctor a person should see. This doctor or nurse practitioner looks at the entire patient and helps navigate the complex medical system. They examine a person, recommend routine screening tests, and write prescriptions for medications when needed. For example, they might write a prescription for antibiotics if a person has a sinus infection.

Specialist doctors involved with cancer include oncologists, radiologists, pathologists and surgeons. Oncologists are specialists in cancer treatments and use medicine, including chemotherapy, to treat cancer. Surgical oncologists and surgeons perform surgery to diagnose and remove the cancers. Radiology oncologists use therapeutic radiation to treat cancer.

Pathologists study the tissue removed during surgery and can identify cancer cells. The information pathologists provide helps guide the other specialists as they recommend the treatments to patients. For example, a surgeon would remove a skin cancer from a person's arm. A pathologist will study the tissue removed, using a microscope, and identify the type of cancer cell and whether the edges of skin (margins) are free of cancer or not. Depending on the pathology findings, the patient might be sent home to heal the surgical incision without any further treatment being needed. If the skin cancer was a slow growing type and was removed, the doctors might recommend only follow-up examinations in the future. If the skin cancer was found to be an aggressive malignant melanoma, the person would be sent for further treatment.

Stages of the Disease

"Staging" refers to the extent or spread of the cancer and doctors consider staging important when recommending treatment. The size of the tumor and whether it has spread to any other area of the body are two key factors in staging. A small cancer insitu (meaning the doctors believe it's only at the one site and has not spread) has a better prognosis (predicted outcome) than a large cancer that has spread and affects other parts of the body.

Several different staging systems are available for doctors to use, so the surgeon or oncologist should explain it so a patient and the family understand what stage the cancer is and what the recommended treatment involves.

Treatments

Treatments for cancer include surgery, radiation, chemotherapy, hormones, and biotherapy. Surgery is the original option, and for many years it was the only option for cancer treatment. During surgery, the cancer is removed if possible. A small, solid tumor can be removed and the patient cured. If however, the cancer has invaded vital organs, removal may be impossible. A biopsy of cancer cells may be taken for diagnosis, and staging and planning for other treatments will begin.

Newer surgical techniques such as cryosurgery, laser surgery, and laparoscopic procedures may help patients recover more quickly and more easily. For example, during cryosurgery, liquid nitrogen treats a tumor which might be in the liver or prostate. Use of a laser beam might be used on a tumor of the vocal cords. Laparoscopic surgery uses small portals, telescopic cameras and instruments to aid the surgeon as he works inside the abdomen. When appropriate, this less invasive procedure would be a quicker, easier recovery for the person undergoing surgery.

Radiation Therapy

C. Kip Bennett went through radiation treatment for his tonsil cancer. Kip says, "It involved them making a mask out of a wicker type device (like a wicker basket) and they wet it so that it shrunk to the size of my face so that during the time I had radiation, not only could I not move; I could barely swallow. They didn't want me moving a bit. They had the computer directing the beam of radiation, which is a huge part of the success of that procedure. Without doing horrific amounts of collateral damage is the way I would describe it, that was the process. With massive doses of radiation, they burned the tonsils out from the outside."

Radiation therapy uses special X-ray machines such as a linear accelerator or a cobalt-60 machine to send radioactive waves or particles into the tissue being treated. Another type treatment occurs when a radioactive substance is given orally or intravenously. For example, iodine (Iodine-131) is taken by mouth as a treatment for thyroid cancer. The use of radioactive beads inserted into tissue or a body cavity is called brachytherapy and gives off radiation to the surrounding tissues. The radiation is emitted for a short time frame and radiation affects both malignant cells and normal cells. Kip remembers Houston cancer doctors telling him they used "a sledgehammer to kill a gnat. Twenty years from now we will look back and say this treatment was barbaric. However, we know how to do it and we're saving lives." Doctors expect treatment to be different in the future.

Side effects can result from injury to normal cells. Tissues most often affected are the skin, mucosa of the GI tract and bone marrow. Side effects include hair falling out, sunburn and skin discoloration and damage. Gastrointestinal symptoms include lack of appetite (anorexia), nausea, vomiting and diarrhea. Fatigue is common. As with chemotherapy, radiation can affect bone marrow function with resulting anemia (decreased white blood cells) and decreased platelets. Lab work for blood counts will probably be done frequently to monitor bone marrow function.

Chemotherapy

Chemotherapy (many people say chemo) refers to drugs used to kill the cancer cells at the cellular level and can be used alone or in combination with other treatments. Chemotherapy drugs can be taken through several methods, including by mouth, and by intravenous shot or infusion at a doctor's office or clinic. Chemotherapy drugs have a specific mechanism of working. For example, methotrexate, one chemotherapy drug, interferes with DNA synthesis of cell reproduction. Other chemotherapy drugs work in different ways.

Which drug will be recommended for a person with lung cancer? Which will be best for leukemia? Researchers have learned much about how different drugs affect cancer cells and which drug or treatment is best for each type of cancer. A personalized plan will be made for each patient during the early days of cancer treatment. In an effort to destroy the cancer cells, a combination of chemotherapy drugs may be recommended. In this situation, drugs with different mechanisms attack the cancer cells in multiple ways and work together in efforts to cure the person.

Chemotherapy drugs attack cells which multiply rapidly (cancer cells). The goal of treatment is to destroy the cancer cells while leaving normal, healthy cells intact. However, many of the chemotherapy drugs are toxic to the normal cells and side effects can occur. A person and family should ask about side effects from the treatments and be prepared to deal with side effects.

Most chemotherapy drugs suppress bone marrow production of blood cells, which results in anemia, neutropenia and thrombocytopenia. Anemia is a low red blood cell count, which explains why a person feels tired, becomes fatigued easily, and is short of breath with exertion. Neutropenia means a low number of neutrophils, one type of white blood cell. Neutropenia explains why a person undergoing chemotherapy faces an increased risk of infection. Thrombocytopenia is an abnormally low number of platelets (blood cells which help form blood clots), which means an increased risk of bleeding.

Another common side effect is nausea, vomiting and anorexia (lack of appetite). Powerful antinausea drugs have been developed in an effort to control this side effect. Another side effect is hair loss (alopecia). Usually the hair will grow back when the drug therapy is completed. However, a person may find it to be traumatic when his hair falls out.

Many chemotherapy drugs are toxic and should be disposed of in special containers. Family and caregivers for persons receiving chemotherapy at home should be given instructions on how to safely dispose of chemotherapy drugs and all containers to protect other family members from any residual drugs.

Hormone Therapy

Hormone therapy involves cancers, such as those of the breast, prostate or endometrium, that are dependent on hormones. For example, a man who has prostate cancer may undergo surgery, an orchiectomy, to remove the testicles and hormones produced by testicles. Then hormonal therapy creates an environment hostile to these cancer cells.

Biotherapy

Biotherapy changes a person's cellular response to better fight cancer. Immunotherapy boosts a person's immune system to recognize cancer cells and fight against them. Passive immunotherapy drugs, such as monoclonal antibodies, use antibodies (or in some cases small fragments of antibodies) to stimulate a patient's immune system to fight cancer cells.

Targeted therapy brings new treatments amid much research and involves attacking the inner working of the cancer cells to disrupt and destroy them while leaving the body's normal cells healthy. One type of targeted therapy, enzyme inhibitors, works because these drugs block specific enzymes that tell cancer cells to grow. Another type, apoptosis-inducing (cell death) drugs, change proteins and cause death within the cancer cells. A third type of drug, called angiogenesis inhibitors, fights cancer by limiting the new blood vessels that some tumors cause to grow as a new blood supply. New treatments and ongoing research can be accessed at the American Cancer Society at www.cancer.org.

Seventy percent of people going through cancer treatment use complementary and alternative therapies.[9] Which therapies are safe and helpful to people dealing with cancer treatments? The American Cancer Society offers advice in their *Complete Guide to Complementary and Alternative Cancer Therapies.*

Prevention Strategies (Risk Factors)

Because lung cancer ranks as the leading cause of death from cancer in both men and women, the experts recommend some lifestyle changes to decrease the risk of lung cancer: Don't smoke or breathe second-hand smoke and reduce exposure to air pollution and cancer-causing substances (carcinogens). The number of Americans who smoke has decreased over the last 40 years (from 42 percent of the population in 1965 to 21 percent in 2009). However, more than 46 million Americans (24 percent of men and 18 percent of women) still smoked in 2009. While nicotine found in the cigarettes is addictive, it's other chemicals found in the tar which cause the most harm. Cigarette smoke contains harmful chemicals such as cyanide, benzene, formaldehyde, methanol or wood alcohol, ammonia, nitrogen oxide and carbon monoxide. The American Cancer Society states "tobacco use accounts for at least 30% of all cancer deaths in the United States. Smoking causes about 87% of lung cancer deaths."[10]

Being overweight increases the risk of cancer of the breast, colon, endometrium, esophagus, kidney and other organs. The ACS recommends a body mass index (BMI) calculator, which can be used to calculate a person's BMI at http://www.cancer.org/Healthy/ToolsandCalculators/Calculators/bodymasscalculator.

When a person types in his height and weight, the calculator will figure his BMI. A BMI below 18.5 is underweight. 18.5 to 24.9 is normal weight; 25 to 29.9 is overweight; 30 and higher is obese. For those whose BMI exceeds a normal weight, the ACS recommends watching portion size and writing down for a few days what and how much is consumed.

When a person analyzes these notes, he may see where he can decrease portion size and cut down on calorie-laden foods.

The American Cancer Society recommends a healthy diet that includes at least five servings of fruits and vegetables (including legumes) and three servings of whole grains daily. They also recommend that people eat less red meat such as beef, lamb and pork, and fewer processed meats such as lunch meat, bologna and hot dogs. Whole grains foods such as whole wheat breads and pastas and brown rice are considered more healthy than white bread, white pasta and white rice. "Being active helps reduce your cancer risk by helping with weight control. It can also help improve your hormone levels and the way your immune system works."[11] The experts recommend a minimum of 30 minutes of exercise daily.

Everyone should protect their skin from the sun. The UVA and UVB rays in sunlight are believed to cause premature aging and skin cancer. Prevention behaviors include covering up, wearing a hat, using a sunscreen and avoiding the intense midday sun. A person's clothing can help protect from UV rays. The experts at the American Cancer Society tell us the best protection comes from wearing long-sleeved pants or skirts, and long-sleeved shirts of dark colors. Loosely woven fabrics of light colors do not protect as well as tightly woven, dark colored clothes. Sun-protective fabrics are being manufactured which add protection from the sun. These clothes will be labeled with the sun-protection factor (SPF). A shirt or pair of pants with an SPF of 50 will protect better than an SPF of 15.

A hat with a wide brim (2 to 3 inches) helps protect the areas most exposed to the sun. A person who wears baseball caps needs to wear sunscreen to protect areas not covered, such as the ears and the neck area. Straw hats should be tightly woven or they won't provide good protection from the sun. Sunscreen needs to be at least an SPF of 30. A higher number increases the protection. "When using an SPF 30 sunscreen and applying it thickly, you get the equivalent of 1 minute of UVB (ultraviolet B) rays for each 30 minutes you spend in the sun. So, 1 hour in the sun wearing SPF 30 sunscreen is the same as spending 2 minutes totally unprotected."[12] SPF 30 sunscreens filter out 97 percent of the UVB rays, while an SPF 50 sunscreen filters out 98 percent of those rays. Currently, sunscreen products are labeled for UVB ray protection only. New guidelines to require labeling of UVA protection is expected in the future. If a sunscreen is labeled "broad-spectrum," it probably provides at least some of both UVB and UVA protection.

To apply sunscreen properly, follow directions by applying it generously (a palmful) to dry, exposed skin such as face, ears, hands, arms and legs. Read and follow the label on the product being used. A general recommendation includes reapplying sunscreen every 2 hours at a minimum and more often if a person is sweating or swimming.

Some sunscreens may irritate an individual's skin. Hypoallergenic products are available. The recommended test is to apply a small amount to the skin of the inner surface of the elbow for 3 days. Discontinue usage if skin irritation, redness, itching or tenderness occurs. Sunscreen has an expiration date and loses its ability to protect after two to three years, so outdated sunscreen should be discarded and new product purchased.

Sunglasses can block UV rays and protect the eyes. Sunglasses which block 99 percent to 100 percent of UVA and UVB rays protect the eyes best. When buying sunglasses, one should look for labels with the words "UV absorption up to 400 nm" or "Meets ANSI UV Requirements." Both these labels indicate UV protection of 99 percent or more. Larger frames and wraparound glasses help protect the eyes from different angles. Sunglasses can be dark or light and still provide UV protection if the invisible protection layer was added during manufacture. Anyone purchasing sunglasses should look for the ANSI label.

Adults caring for children and young people should be protecting them from sun rays by covering them up, using appropriate sunscreen on them, and limiting their exposure to the sun. Their eyes should be protected by smaller versions of real sunglasses with UV protection. The American Cancer Society makes this recommendation: "You should develop the habit of using sunscreen on exposed skin for yourself and your children whenever you go outdoors and may be exposed to large amounts of sunlight. If you or your child burns easily, be extra careful to cover up, limit exposure, and apply sunscreen. Babies younger than 6 months should be kept out of direct sunlight and protected from the sun using hats and protective clothing."[13] The most intense sunlight and UV rays occur during the middle of the day, usually between 10 A.M. and 4 P.M. Staying inside during those hours helps one limit exposure to UV rays. Beware of cloudy days when it's easy to stay out in the sun longer and not recognize the increased amount of UV rays you are getting. UV rays pass through clouds. Reapply the sunscreen even on cloudy, comfortable-temperature days to avoid overexposure to the sun. Also, sand and snow reflect the sun and can compound the effects of the rays, so extra protection should be used on the beach and around snow.

Tanning beds aren't recommended: "Tanning lamps give out UVA and usually UVB rays as well. Both UVA and UVB rays can cause serious long-term skin damage, and can contribute to skin cancer."[14]

Research

The earliest recorded case of cancer was in Egypt back in 1600 B.C. Hippocrates (460 to 370 B.C.), the "Father of Medicine," coined the word cancer. Many physicians over the centuries have observed the disease and cared for people dealing with it. In 1962, Nobel Prize winners James Watson and Francis Crick identified DNA (deoxyribonucleic acid), the genetic information in cells. Since that time, research continues as scientists work to identify the causes of cancers and what preventive measures work and don't work. Doctors look at how treatments save lives and what can be done to improve the treatments. Researchers around the world strive to find cures for the over 100 different types of cancer and the people dealing with them.

Caregivers and the Disease

An advocate is necessary for a person undergoing cancer treatments. As Kip said, "It became pretty obvious to me as a patient that you tend to over focus on some of the things that catch your attention. The more horrific they are, the more likely you are to hit the bottom of your boat there and you stop. The doctor goes on and you miss the next ten things he says, nine of which are very important. Having someone there who is a little more emotionally detached from the circumstance and can write down or help you think back on what he (the medical professional) said is really important. Get someone to go with you is my message on that."[15]

The advocate/caregiver should get contact phone numbers for the different doctors' offices to access the help needed. If the person undergoing chemotherapy needs medication for nausea, having phone numbers will simplify getting help. Support groups can help a person and family who are dealing with cancer and treatments. The American Cancer Society offers the Cancer Survivors Network at http://www.cancer.org/treatment/supportprogramsservices.index as an online support.

Emotions can be challenging for a person dealing with cancer. Anxiety and fear often begin when a person knows "something is wrong." These emotions become constant companions throughout the treatments and even afterwards. Small changes in a person's body, for example a sore which won't heal after radiation treatment, can strike fear in the person and his family. More doctor appointments and tests may be needed to answer the question of whether the cancer is back. This roller coaster of emotions can be challenging for the patient and his loved ones.

Family and caring friends can bring support to a person undergoing treatments. At one point, Kip recognized his will to go on was exhausted. He invited his entire family to his lake property for the weekend and he planned to say good-bye to them. During the course of the weekend, he was doing just that — talking to each person. At one point, Kip's 27-year-old son, Eric, asked, "Dad, will you help me tether the boat?" Kip said he told him, "I'm busy, you do it." Eric again asked, "Dad, would you please come help me tie up the boat?" Kip said, "Ok, but you are interrupting my plans. You can tie up the boat by yourself." Kip followed his son down to the dock and his son reached out and hugged him. Eric said, "Whether you die or I die, we cannot change what happens to us. But it bothers me a lot that you aren't going to the place I plan to spend eternity. I want you to start going to church with me."

Kip continued: "There were Sundays that I literally laid on the pew during church and took a nap because I was so exhausted from the treatments. But every Sunday my son took me to church. Now I try to make the most of every day.... I re–examined my priorities after this conversation with my son."

Caring medical providers can support those undergoing cancer treatments. Kip relates this story, which happened after all his treatments were finished and he was home. Side effects to his radiation treatment involved difficulty swallowing and increased mucus or saliva. He would get dehydrated and have to go to his local hospital for rehydration through intravenous fluids.

One night he was admitted to the nursing unit for intravenous fluids. This night the area was quiet, too quiet, and Kip found himself asking the nurse taking care of him to please sit with him. "I was afraid to close my eyes. I didn't have much faith that I would wake up." That nurse sat with him while she charted. After she finished, she gently scratched his arm until he relaxed and fell asleep. Kip remembers her compassionate care that night: "I was afraid for my life. I didn't want to say that to people but that was what was on my mind. She was one of the people who got it."

C. Kip Bennett shares these thoughts: "You just have to know you're going to have some hard times to get to the other side (a cure). Getting up everyday and making coffee certainly is its own reward. But it's not just being alive, the quality of my life is so much better after having the procedure of choice."[16]

14

Diabetes

Katie Bond's world turned upside down. Pete, her husband of sixty-plus years, had been trying to get well after a bout of pneumonia but couldn't. He ate Thanksgiving Day dinner at daughter Sue Wessel's home and went for a nap which lasted much longer than usual. The long nap caused his family concern as they realized that Pete was very ill. Within a couple days, Pete entered the hospital. Despite antibiotics, breathing treatments and all efforts by doctors and family over a six-week period, Pete never returned home to Katie. He succumbed to his illness and died.

What was Katie to do? She didn't want to return home where she had lived with Pete and raised their children; there were too many memories. Her family did not want Katie to live alone. At age 86, Katie deals with various ailments including osteoporosis. Fortunately for Katie, her loving family had planned for this day. Daughter Jan and her husband, Bob Gile, were building a new home complete with a "mother-in-law" suite. They invited Katie to move in with them and she did. Everyone adjusted to a new routine. Katie lives with Bob and Jan the majority of the time but she often goes to the home of daughter Sue and her husband, Jack Wessel, for extended stays. With the help of her family, Katie dealt with her grief and fragile health.

It was over a year later that Katie was diagnosed with diabetes. Even Katie's doctor was surprised that Katie's blood sugar was elevated. She had gone to the doctor for a routine checkup. Daughter Jan recalls, "We took mom for a six month check up on her blood pressure medicine. I had noticed that her bedside commode contained urine that was cloudy in appearance. Mom has a history of frequent urinary tract infections (UTI). I told Mom's doctor, 'I think she has been going to the bathroom more frequently; she might have a UTI.' The doctor said, 'Let's do some lab work; it's been a while since she had any done....' The next day the doctor's office called with this message: 'We need to talk about your mom's blood results.' We took Mom back into the doctor's office for this report: Mom's blood sugar (not fasting) was 439, her A1C was 12.1 and her urine had 3–4 plus sugar."[1]

Daughter Sue shared this: "It was a shock because I didn't realize it could be happening for my mom. Often the people who have diabetes are overweight or obese. Mom weighs 100 pounds. Most of the time diabetes patients are younger in age.... I was taken aback by it."[2] Daughter Jan immediately felt bad: "She lives with us. We're both medical; I'm a nurse and my husband is an anesthesiologist. Why didn't we pick up on it?"

Katie's doctor was just as surprised as anyone. He told them type 2 diabetes often comes on slowly; they should not feel guilty about not recognizing the diabetes. He started Katie on 2mg of an oral diabetes medication called Amaryl. He said he wanted to see Katie again in 3 weeks for a recheck and that he might need to raise her Amaryl dosage. He felt it wise to monitor her blood sugar and make adjustments in her medicine slowly.

The first step for Katie's family was learning about her type 2 diabetes. Within a week Katie, Jan, Sue and Katie's caregiver were all attending diabetes education classes taught by a dietitian and a nurse. They learned how to operate Katie's new glucose meter and how to test her blood sugar. The dietitian explained the 1500 calorie diet and how to count carbohydrates. Katie's recommended 12 servings of carbohydrates per day meant the daughters needed to read labels on food packages.

Sue says, "Labels are easy to read.... I did gain a lot when we went to diabetic education and met with the nurse and dietitian. I was really concerned but a lot of it was common sense." Jan agrees the diabetic education was valuable. They "found Mom can have more foods than we realized. It's important for a diabetic person to have appropriate snacks. I tell Mom's caregiver to be sure Mom has a snack around 2–3 P.M. I always make sure Mom has a snack before she goes to bed at night.... Also Medicare will pay for a certain amount of teaching the first year (from a dietitian and a diabetic education nurse) and additional diabetic teaching after that. They were excellent."

Diabetes Mellitus — What Is It?

"Diabetes mellitus is a group of diseases marked by high levels of blood glucose resulting from defects in insulin production, insulin action, or both."[3]

Type 1 diabetes mellitus (also called insulin-dependent diabetes mellitus or IDDM) occurs when the pancreas does not make insulin. The pancreas cannot make insulin because its insulin-producing cells, called pancreatic beta cells, have been destroyed. A person with Type 1 diabetes must take insulin shots (either by injection or insulin pump) to regulate his blood sugar. This form of diabetes may be caused by autoimmune disease, environmental damage or inherited causes. Type 1 diabetes can happen at any age, but most often strikes children and young adults and accounts for only 5 percent to 10 percent of all diagnosed cases of diabetes in adults.

Type 2 diabetes mellitus (also called non-insulin-dependent diabetes mellitus or NIDDM) happens when the body cells cannot use the insulin the pancreas produces (insulin resistance) or the pancreas doesn't produce enough insulin. Type 2 diabetes often begins as insulin resistance and progresses to the condition where the pancreas cannot produce enough insulin. Risk factors for type 2 diabetes include older age, obesity, family history of diabetes, a history of gestational diabetes (during pregnancy), impaired glucose metabolism, physical inactivity and race/ethnicity. People at risk because of race/ethnicity include African Americans, Hispanic American, American Indians and some Asian/Hawaiian Americans. Type 2 accounts for 90 to 95 percent of all diagnosed cases of diabetes.

Who Gets Diabetes?

In America, 23.6 million people (7.8 percent of the population) have diabetes mellitus. 17.9 million are diagnosed and 5.7 million people have undiagnosed diabetes mellitus."[4]

Symptoms

The classic symptoms of diabetes mellitus are constant thirst and drinking of water (polydipsia), excessive urination (polyuria) and excessive hunger (polyphagia). These symptoms occur because the high blood sugar level forces the kidneys to work harder to rid the body of the excess blood sugar. The person urinates more often (polyuria) and becomes dehydrated and is thirsty (polydipsia). When excessive hunger (polyphagia) occurs, it's because the person's body can't utilize the blood sugar efficiently. The cells don't get the sugar they need from the blood because the insulin can't help transport the sugar into the cell. Other symptoms include unexplained weight loss, fatigue, infections and blurred vision.

In hindsight, Katie's symptoms were masked and easily explained. Sue Wessel shares these thoughts: "Diabetic patients are always thirsty and Mom was always drinking water but that was a norm for her. She has always been a good water drinker even way back so that didn't ring a bell. Yes, she liked her sweets. That wasn't unusual for her.... Now that we look back, a lot of these symptoms had to do with her sugars because she had no energy. But she has osteoporosis and uses a walker. We attributed that to her age; at 80 plus years she's not going to run circles."

Important Structures and What Happens

The pancreas is a six-inch long organ found in the upper left side of the abdomen (behind the stomach). It makes pancreatic juices and hormones including insulin and glucagon. The pancreatic juices are released into the small intestine where they help digest food.

Both insulin and glucagon are produced by the islets of Langerhans area of the pancreas. Insulin is produced by beta cells. "The release of insulin from the pancreatic beta cells is regulated by blood glucose (sugar) levels, increasing as blood glucose levels rise and decreasing when blood glucose levels decline."[5] In other words, the pancreas releases insulin when blood sugar levels are high. Insulin enables the body to move sugar carried in the blood into cells where it's used for energy or stored. "Only insulin has the effect of lowering the blood glucose level."[6]

Glucagon is produced by alpha cells of the pancreas and functions in an opposite manner to insulin. "As with insulin, glucagon secretion is regulated by blood glucose. A decrease in blood glucose concentration to a hypoglycemic level (low blood sugar) produces an immediate increase in glucagon secretion, and an increase in blood glucose to hyperglycemic levels (high blood sugar) produces a decrease in glucagon secretion."[7] Glucagon is released when blood sugar levels are low and stimulates the body to break down stored reserves to raise blood sugar to normal levels. Both insulin and glucagon are released into the blood stream in the body's efforts to regulate blood sugar levels. Other hormones are involved but insulin and glucagon are the major hormones that regulate blood sugar levels.

Nutrition

To understand the significance of high blood sugar, one must understand some basic nutrition. Nutrition is the breakdown of food providing energy and nutrients the body needs to be healthy.

The three main nutrients in food are carbohydrates, lipids (fats), and proteins. From these nutrients, a person's body pulls energy. A person eats a meal and the body begins its work of breaking down the nutrients. The bonds between the nutrients' atoms break. "As the bonds break, they release energy. Some of this energy is released as heat, but some is used to send electrical impulses through the brain and nerves, to synthesize body compounds, and to move muscles. Thus the energy from food supports every activity from quiet thought to vigorous sports."[8]

The word "carbs" brings to mind pastas, rice and bread. As a group of nutrients, carbohydrates are made of three simple sugars (glucose, fructose and galactose). Glucose is the easy-to-use energy source for the human body. More complex carbohydrates (disaccharides and complex carbohydrates such as starches) are combinations of these simple sugars. The body is able to use simple sugars quickly, while more complex carbohydrates require more time and energy to break down (metabolize) into the simple sugars. Starches (grains) include rice, wheat, corn, barley, rye, oats, legumes and tubers such as potatoes and yams.

Carbohydrates are broken down into a simple sugar (most often glucose) which acts as a major fuel source. Normally a person's body releases insulin, which helps the body cells pull glucose from the blood. Body cells then utilize this sugar as energy. A person's brain and nervous system must have glucose from the blood to do its work. Glucose must be available in the blood almost constantly because the brain and nervous system can't make glucose or store more than a few minutes' supply of it. This explains why low blood sugar results in a person's inability to concentrate and symptoms of headache, dizziness or confusion.

When a person eats more than the body uses, the excess glucose is stored as glycogen in the liver or turned to fat (adipose tissue). Later in the day that person is busy and can't get to a snack. He's feeling hungry, his stomach is grumbling, and his blood glucose level lowers. The body converts the stored glucose (glycogen) back into glucose and constantly balances its need for glucose and the storage of excess glucose as glycogen in the liver and muscle cells.

The second major nutrient is lipids (also called fats). The human body needs lipids as a second energy source. Many portions of the body, but not the brain and nervous system, can use fats as energy. Lipids also benefit a person by providing the basis for hormones, vitamin D and bile. The body's stored fats provide insulation from temperature extremes and act as a shock absorber for body organs.

When a person eats a large meal, the unused fats are transported through the blood as triglycerides. As triglycerides travel past adipose cells, an enzyme on the surface of the adipose cell grabs the triglyceride out of the bloodstream, breaks it down into fatty acids and stores it. Later the body needs energy from the fatty acids. An enzyme inside the adipose cells breaks down the stored fat, converts it into smaller compounds and energy and releases them into the bloodstream. When body fat is broken down in the absence of carbohydrates, small fragments of fat are not metabolized and ketone bodies result. A build-up of ketone bodies in the blood can result in ketoacidosis, a life-threatening complication for a person with type 1 diabetes.

The third main food nutrient is proteins. Proteins, made up of amino acids, are important building blocks for the muscles, bone, genes, hemoglobin part of red blood cells and skin cells of the body. Proteins are important components of hormones such as insulin, glucagon and growth hormone. The body uses proteins as key ingredients in enzymes, antibodies, and transport molecules. When a person eats more protein than needed, only a limited amount can be stored. The excess protein is converted into fatty acids, glucose and ketones.

A person's digestive system, including the liver, breaks down food (whether carbohydrates, fats or proteins) into a usable form. The carbohydrates are broken down into glucose. The fats are broken down into fatty acids. Proteins are broken down into amino acids.

When a person's blood sugar becomes low between meals, glucagon is released by the pancreas, and the body turns glycogen back into glucose. When blood sugar is high from a recent meal, the pancreas releases insulin, which enables the body cells to pull sugar from the blood and use the sugar for energy. When the body no longer can control the blood sugar on its own, that person finds himself dealing with diabetes. The good news is that people can practice healthy lifestyle behaviors and avoid or delay the complications of diabetes.

Diagnosis

Diagnosis of diabetes mellitus is made after a laboratory test which shows an elevated blood sugar. The lab test Katie Bond's doctor ordered is called a casual blood glucose test because it can be drawn at any time whether a person has eaten or not. When the casual blood glucose test results are above 200 mg/dL and a person has symptoms consistent with diabetes (polydipsia, polyuria, polyphagia, and blurred vision), a diagnosis of diabetes mellitus is made. Katie's casual blood glucose test result was 439.

Two other lab tests which a doctor may prescribe is a fasting plasma glucose test (FPG) and an oral glucose tolerance test (OGTT). A fasting plasma (or blood) glucose test involves blood being drawn after a person fasts (no food) for 8 to 12 hours. An FPG result of less than 100 mg/dL is normal. An FPG result between 100 and 125 mg/dL is borderline (impaired fasting glucose or prediabetes) and A FPG result above 126 mg/dL is considered positive for diabetes mellitus.

An OGTT measures how efficiently the body handles glucose. A person should be fasting for several hours before the first blood test is obtained at the laboratory. The person then drinks a sugar drink (a specific amount of concentrated glucose.) The lab test continues as blood samples are obtained to measure the blood sugar levels at specific time frames. The doctor expects that a person with diabetes mellitus would have higher blood glucose levels which remain high longer than a person who is not diabetic. Results of the OGTT are as follows: Less than 140 mg/dL is considered a normal result; a result of 140–199 mg/dL is considered prediabetes; a result above 200 mg/dL is considered diabetes mellitus.[9]

The A1C (glycated hemoglobin) test is a blood test which measures the blood glucose levels for the past 12 weeks. The rationale behind this test involves how much glucose (sugar) attaches to hemoglobin of the red blood cells. Hemoglobin (the oxygen carrying part of the red blood cells) lives 120 days and does not contain glucose when it's released into the bloodstream. As the hemoglobin portion of the red blood cells circulates through the bloodstream, glucose permanently attaches to it. When a person's blood sugar (glucose) level is elevated, this will show up in an A1C blood test. According to the American Diabetes Association, the goal for a person's A1C is below 7 percent.[10] Katie Bond's initial A1C blood test was 12.1 percent at the time she was diagnosed with type 2 diabetes mellitus. Her most recent A1C blood test report was 7.2 percent.

Self Testing of Blood Sugar

A person with either type 1 or type 2 diabetes needs to learn how to check his blood sugar and expect this to be a routine part of life. A periodic A1C test will not replace routine self testing of blood sugar. A person's doctor will recommend how often that person should check his blood sugar. For some people, once daily will be sufficient. For others, especially newly diagnosed diabetics and type 1 diabetics using insulin, self-testing may need to be done several times throughout the day.

A person will be taught how to monitor his blood sugar using a blood glucose meter. To prevent infection, a person should wash his hands with soap and water or an alcohol swab, allow the finger to dry, then prick the side of the finger and squeeze a drop of blood onto the blood glucose monitor strip. The glucose meter "reads" the blood sugar level on the strip and numbers appear in the display window of the meter. The recommended site of obtaining blood and operation of the monitor will vary according to the glucose meter. The diabetes education nurse will teach a patient and his family how to do self-testing and will also answer any questions they might have.

Finding the Right Doctor

Most people find their family doctor/primary care physician able to provide the care they need while dealing with diabetes mellitus. If their diabetes is difficult to control, their primary care physician may refer them to an endocrinologist, a medical doctor with additional training to deal with diabetes and other hormone related conditions.

Prediabetes and Preventing the Development of Diabetes Type 2

Prediabetes means a person's body can't handle glucose properly. This person is at risk for developing type 2 diabetes and its complications. A doctor would talk about prediabetes to the patient whose fasting plasma sugar (FPS) is elevated to between 100 and 125 mg/dL. This person's blood sugar is elevated but not to the numbers considered diabetic (126 mg/dL and higher). The other common indicator for prediabetes involves a slightly elevated result to a 2-hour oral glucose tolerance test. If a person's OGTT result was between 140 and 199 mg/dL, his doctor would talk to this person about prediabetes risks.

Experts estimate that 79 million Americans have prediabetes, a borderline high blood sugar level,[11] and face an increased risk of developing type 2 diabetes. Can these people prevent or at least delay the onset of diabetes? Doctors say yes. The person with prediabetes faces an opportunity to improve his health. "Studies have shown that people with prediabetes who lose weight and increase their physical activity can prevent or delay diabetes and return their blood glucose levels to normal."[12] Recommended behavior changes include losing excess weight, moving more (increasing physical activity) and changing one's eating habits. A person should talk with his doctor for recommendations about losing weight and taking up exercise. It sounds simple: use more calories than one eats. However, many people battle this situation. The other recommendation (beginning to exercise) also contributes positive changes to the goal of preventing diabetes and losing weight.

Doctors Roizen and Oz give their opinion on the role of exercise in preventing diabetes: "The most important things you can do to lower your risk of diabetes are to keep your waist thin, exercise (thirty minutes daily), and keep your blood pressure under control.... A little physical activity can dramatically improve the ability of insulin to get glucose into many cells, especially muscle."[13] Researchers believe that physical activity helps the body utilize insulin more effectively. In addition, exercise revs up a person's metabolism, burns calories and helps him better deal with stress. The National Institutes of Health recommends 30 minutes of exercise 5 days a week. Some easy ways to add exercise include parking the car farther away from work or stores and walking to the building and taking TV commercial time to walk around the house or do exercises. One group of women walk during their 30 minute lunchtime after they eat. A person can add exercise by walking the stairs instead of using the elevator.[14]

A harried caregiver may feel the need to hurry home and check on Mom; 30 minutes a day for exercise is too much time for an overcrowded schedule. However, this caregiver may find she can squeeze three ten minute walks into her schedule. If she parks farther away from her work building and walks, she can get exercise. She can eat lunch and then use 10 or 15 minutes of her lunch hour for a short walk. Gardening or housecleaning chores done during the evening hours can contribute to her exercise time. Benefit is gained from exercise both physically and mentally.

A person can improve his eating habits by making some easy changes. One can add color to his plate by adding a variety of fruits and vegetables.

Colorful foods add vitamins and minerals to a person's diet. One can substitute whole grain foods (more complex carbohydrates) for refined foods. Brown rice is a more healthy choice than white rice. Whole grain pastas and breads fit into a healthy diet. One can lower fat intake by baking or broiling foods instead of frying. Another way to lower fat intake is by using nonfat and low-fat foods (for example, fat-free milk instead of whole milk). Other healthy changes happen when one drinks water instead of sugared sodas and soft drinks and switches to healthy snacks such as raw vegetables and fruits. All these suggested behaviors are recommended for a person with prediabetes who wants to prevent or delay moving into diabetes.[15]

Treatment of Diabetes

Once a person is diagnosed with either type 1 or type 2 diabetes, he will need glucose control. Controlling a person's blood sugar helps decrease complications: "Every percentage point drop in A1c blood test results (e.g., from 8.0 percent to 7.0 percent) can reduce the risk of microvascular complications (eye, kidney and nerve diseases) by 40 percent."[16]

Treatment of type 1 diabetes involves insulin, and the type 1 person will need insulin replacement by injection or insulin pump.

Individuals dealing with type 2 diabetes have more options. For one person, lifestyle changes such as managing meals, losing weight, and exercising brings the blood sugar under control and medication won't be needed. This person can learn how to read labels and by controlling carbohydrate intake, he can control his blood sugar. For other individuals, treatment means oral diabetes medication or possibly insulin. Each person dealing with diabetes should be instructed on medications and proper administration of this medication. The doctor, pharmacist, and diabetes education staff can provide personalized information. Diabetes education should be step one in learning about a healthy lifestyle and a personalized food plan. Attending classes held by a dietitian and a diabetes education nurse will answer questions and bring the newly diagnosed person into a "can do" attitude.

Katie's family benefited from the diabetes education. Daughter Sue Wessel had this to say:

> Once you learn what a diabetic can have, it's not hard. Now Mom uses sugar free syrup so that's easy. There's so much out there that fits a sugar free diet that wasn't available in years past. What I don't understand is why sugar free

foods are more expensive but I guess it's because they use the sugar substitute instead of sugar. It's sad; we can afford to buy Mother's food but I feel bad for people who are diabetics who have to go to the grocery store and can only afford a sugar free cookie every now and then instead of having them more often. They're going to pay more for a sugar free cookie than a regular cookie. My husband and I try to watch what we eat too so it's probably been good for us.

A personalized plan from a doctor will address how often a person's blood sugar should be monitored. Katie's blood sugar is currently monitored once daily. At the beginning, her daughters checked her blood sugar several times a day, trying to establish a pattern. Daughter Jan shares this information: "One thing I found out the hard way, Medicare will only pay for one (glucose monitor) strip per day which is fine. But we didn't know that up front." Over a period of several months of monitoring, her medication level has been increased slowly. Jan continued: "The doctor told us he wanted to raise her medication gradually. He did not want to drop her blood sugar too much and risk that at her age, she might get weak, pass out, fall and break a hip or other bone. At her August checkup, the doctor checked her A1C and it was 7.2. He was very pleased."

Katie reports that she's adjusted well. She's feeling better and sleeping better. She said, "I have no objection to what the girls put out for me to eat.... I don't mind taking the medicine."[17] Katie reports she can still have some of her favorite foods such as cottage cheese, ice cream (sugar-free, of course) and peaches.

Preventing Chronic Complications of Diabetes

"Diabetes was the seventh leading cause of death listed on U.S. death certificates in 2006." Overall, diabetes doubles the risk of death compared to people of similar age who don't have diabetes.[18] "Diabetes is a significant risk factor in coronary heart disease and stroke, and it is the leading cause of blindness and chronic kidney disease, as well as a major contributor to lower extremity amputations."[19] Statistics prove that diabetes contributes to kidney disease, heart disease and stroke, high blood pressure, blindness, and neuropathy (nerve damage). "A person with uncontrolled diabetes is unable to transport glucose into fat and muscle cells; as a result, body cells are starved and the breakdown of fat and protein is increased to generate alternative fuels."[20]

The high blood sugar which constantly circulates through a person's bloodstream does harm to the kidneys. The kidneys act as a filter in the body, cleansing the blood of impurities, and also make chemicals which help regulate a person's blood pressure. If blood sugar is high, the kidneys struggle to filter the sugar. This person can experience frequent infections because bacteria thrive in the high sugar content in the blood and urine. The uncontrolled high sugar causes kidney failure. "Diabetes is the leading cause of kidney failure, accounting for 44 percent of new cases in 2005."[21] High blood sugar also damages blood vessels and nerves. Both large blood vessels (macrocirculation) and small blood vessels (microcirculation) are affected. The macrocirculation blood vessels includes coronary (heart), cerebral (brain), vascular and peripheral vascular (arms and legs) arteries.

If we compare people whose blood sugar is high to the general population, we see that diseases of the large blood vessels develop earlier, get worse and are more severe in those with high blood sugar. If the person with diabetes is overweight or obese and has high blood pressure and high blood lipid levels, his risk of vascular disease affecting his heart, brain or peripheral circulation increases even more. A loss of blood supply (a blocked artery) to the heart can cause a heart attack. A stroke could occur if blood supply to the brain is decreased or damaged. When the blood vessels to a person's legs are damaged, the person may experience pain and cold feet which can progress to tissue death and ulcers, requiring a lower leg amputation.

The small blood vessels (microcirculation) involve capillaries in the eyes and kidneys. When compared to the general population, a person who has uncontrolled blood sugars has increased risk of damage in the blood vessels of the eyes (retinopathy) and kidneys (nephropathy): "Diabetic retinopathy is estimated to be the most frequent cause of newly diagnosed blindness among Americans between the ages of 20 and 74 years."[22] The elevated blood sugars cause damage to the eye and can result in blindness.

Uncontrolled blood sugar harms the nerves of the body. The damaged blood vessels means the blood supply to nerves may be inadequate and damage occurs to the nerves. "About 60–70 percent of people with diabetes have mild to severe forms of nervous system damage. The results of such damage include impaired sensation or pain in the feet or hands, slowed digestion of food in the stomach, carpal tunnel syndrome, erective dysfunction, or other nerve problems."[23]

If nerves in the feet are affected, a person may lose sensation there and might not feel the discomfort which would warn him that a sore was developing on the foot. When the sore becomes infected and reddened, he might not recognize the danger until a severe infection threatened the foot. This person could face losing his foot and leg due to a diabetic sore which developed into gangrene.

Doctors believe a controlled blood sugar within normal levels can help prevent or delay these complications of diabetes. Someone suffering with diabetes may get tired of dealing with it. Some people lose their perspective and decide to eat what they want and not work to control their blood sugar. However, they will benefit from working with their medical resources. "In general, every percentage point drop in A1c blood test results (e.g., from 8.0% to 7.0%) can reduce the risk of microvascular complications (eye, kidney and nerve diseases) by 40%."[24]

A person with prediabetes or diabetes type 1 or 2 can work to improve his health by controlling his blood sugar, his blood pressure and his blood lipid (cholesterol) levels. Controlling blood pressure and blood lipid levels contributes to health and helps avoid complications. "For every 10 mm HG reduction in systolic (top number) blood pressure, the risk for any complication related to diabetes is reduced by 12%.... Improved control of LDL (low density lipoprotein) cholesterol can reduce cardiovascular complications by 20 to 50%."[25]

Life-Threatening Complications

Three life-threatening complications can affect a person with diabetes, type 1 or 2: diabetic ketoacidosis, hyperosmolar hyperglycemic state and hypoglycemia. All three complications require hospitalization, careful observation, and appropriate treatments.

Diabetic ketoacidosis occurs when the blood sugar gets too high and ketones and acidosis develop. Diabetic ketoacidosis most often affects those people with type 1 diabetes. When insulin is inadequate, the glucose in the bloodstream cannot enter the cells and they are forced to break down fat to get energy. Ketone bodies result and cause the body to become acidic.

Symptoms of diabetic ketoacidosis include slow, deep breathing, a fruity odor to the breath, confusion, poor appetite, frequent urination and loss of consciousness. Diabetic ketoacidosis can be triggered by infection, physical or emotion stress, anxiety, and pregnancy.[26] The condition is considered a life-threatening emergency. Treatment at a hospital or medical center will be needed to control the person's blood sugar and rehydrate the person and counteract the ketoacidosis.

Hyperosmolar hyperglycemic state (HHS) is a high blood sugar crisis which can affect people with type 2 diabetes. No ketoacidosis occurs, but a high blood sugar causes a serious dehydration within the body which can be life-threatening. Symptoms of HHS include weakness, dehydration, frequent urination, excessive thirst and neurologic symptoms. The neurologic symptoms can mimic a stroke with hemiparesis (one-side weakness), fever, the inability to speak, vision problems, seizures and a coma. Hyperosmolar hyperglycemic state can be triggered by infection, uncontrolled type 2 diabetes, a heart attack, or acute pancreatitis. Treatment of it requires rehydration of the person and control of the blood sugar while the patient's fluid and electrolyte status is monitored.

Hypoglycemia (insulin reaction) occurs when the blood sugar level becomes too low. Hypoglycemia can occur in both type 1 and type 2 diabetes patients. Symptoms of hypoglycemia include headache, difficulty thinking clearly and solve problems. These symptoms (which can progress to seizure and coma) happen because the brain needs glucose. Other symptoms include hunger, anxiety, a fast heart rate, and being cool and clammy. Symptoms may vary a lot among individuals, especially children and the elderly. Hypoglycemia can be triggered by taking too much insulin, exercising more than usual without adjusting food intake and medication levels, failure to eat, or medication changes which change insulin needs.

Treatment of hypoglycemia is to give sugar in some form (glucose or glycogen in a hospital setting). Many type 1 diabetic people learn to pay attention and treat their hypoglycemic symptoms early before they become life-threatening.

Research into Diabetes

Researchers have learned a great deal in recent years. For type 1 diabetes, doctors have transplanted pancreatic islet (beta) cells. For the recipients, the resulting production of insulin brings elation. But the human body wants to reject those transplanted cells and the recipient must take anti-rejection drugs. Is there a better way to handle this situation? Researchers at the Diabetes Research Institute are working to see whether mesenchymal stem cells (MSCs) can accomplish a decreased inflammatory response: "If MSCs can reduce or prevent the inflammation that occurs after transplantation, we can enhance the long-term viability of the islet cells needed to restore natural insulin production.... There's also evidence that MSCs can reverse rejection, which means we may be able to use them to lower the amount of immunosuppression (anti-rejection drugs) that islet transplant patients must now take long term."[27]

What about preventing complications of diabetes? Thanks to past studies like the Diabetes Control and Complications Trial (DCCT) and Epidemiology of Diabetes Interventions and Complications (EDIC) Trial, researchers and doctors believe that a controlled blood sugar enables a person to reap benefits: preventing or at least delaying complications such as eye disease, kidney disease, heart and cardiovascular disease, and nerve disease. These studies involved people who have type 1 diabetes. However, researchers believe the results of the DCCT and EDIC studies are true for people with both type 1 and type 2 diabetes because "the microvascular disease development process is likely to be similar for both type 1 and type 2 diabetes."[28]

What can a person with prediabetes do to avoid developing type 2 diabetes? Researchers at the Diabetes Prevention Program (DPP) found over three years of study that "intensive lifestyle modification reduced the incidence of type 2 diabetes development by 58 percent, while metformin treatment reduced diabetes incidence by 31 percent." A ten year follow-up study found "lifestyle changes including healthy diet and exercise, as well as metformin therapy although to a lesser extent, can decrease the risk of type 2 diabetes by more than one third — even several years after the initial intervention."[29] Ongoing research around the world continues as doctors and researchers search for a better understanding of diabetes, who gets it, how to prevent it and better treatments for those suffering from it.

Caregivers and the Disease

Caregivers may find themselves learning about diabetes in order to care for their loved one. They may begin reading food labels in grocery stores and planning meals for a loved one who has diabetes, or learning how to test blood sugar levels and give insulin shots when they need to do so. Caregivers watch for complications of diabetes. Jan shares this information: "Recently Mom took a fall and scraped her elbow and her shin. I asked her several times, 'Does that hurt?' She said, 'No.' That's a red flag to me. I know with diabetes people lose sensation. It worries me that if it (her shin) would become hot and red, would she notice it doesn't feel good and she's developing an infection? Also when Mom's sugar was high, she would talk about her dentures rubbing and being sore. Her gums were tender. Since we've gotten her sugar under control, Mom has only mentioned one time her dentures being sore."

Caregivers must deal with their own health issues, and for some caregivers that means diabetes. A busy caregiver may not take the time he needs to exercise daily, which would help with controlling his blood sugar level. A busy caregiver may grab fast food because he's tired and hungry as he drives by Mom's house to check on her. Caregivers juggle many responsibilities and may feel their own health can wait. The best outcome for a person dealing with his own diabetes comes when a person keeps his blood sugar under control. By working with his doctor, this caregiver can practice healthy life style behaviors such as exercising, eating healthy foods and monitoring his blood sugar.

Caregivers need to remember the truth in airline safety instructions: if something happens and the oxygen masks drop down, each person must take time to put on his own oxygen mask before trying to help someone else put one on. Caregivers should do the same: care for self first, keep self healthy and then care for the loved one. Both caregiver and care receiver will benefit from this strategy.

15

Heart Disease

Ray began having pressure in his chest, neck and jaw. This 79-year-old man quietly walked to the bedroom and laid across the bed. He was having difficulty catching his breath and he was sweating profusely. After he rested a few minutes, the pain eased up and he fell asleep. When he awakened from the nap, he got up thinking he should finish mowing the lawn. As he began pulling the starter rope, he noticed that pressure again but he persisted. After all, he thought, mowing the lawn was his job. But the pain increased and he found himself sitting on the front porch, gasping to catch his breath when his wife of 54 years, Rebecca, came out to check on him. "What's wrong with you?" she asked.

"I can't catch my breath and I'm having chest pain." No more conversation was necessary. Rebecca flew into the house and called their nurse daughter.

"Mom, call an ambulance and get him to the hospital. He may be having a heart attack. I'll call the girls and we will meet you there."

Within a short time, Ray was taken by ambulance to their local hospital. The family's suspicions were confirmed. Ray had blocked coronary arteries and needed open heart bypass surgery. The doctors offered him few choices: he could have surgery or become a "cardiac cripple" until the blockage caused a fatal heart attack. The family rallied around Ray and Rebecca and encouraged him to have the surgery. Easter Sunday was spent visiting Ray in the cardiac care unit, waiting for the Monday morning surgery. Ray came through the procedure with an excellent prognosis.

No one recognized the toll being placed on Rebecca. After long days sitting in the waiting room to visit Ray and going home exhausted at night, Rebecca called her daughter one night to say, "Please come help me. I can't catch my breath." The daughter raced the few blocks across town to her mother's side. When she arrived, she saw her mother gasping in distress and she could hear the gurgling sounds she made. When the ambulance staff arrived, they immediately started oxygen, monitored her vital signs, and were instructed by the emergency room doctor to give her Lasix. This was Rebecca's first bout with congestive heart failure; she ended up in the progressive coronary care unit at the same hospital. Now the daughters had to tell Dad that Mom was in the hospital and they knew he would start worrying. In the days before cell phones, this challenge was dealt with by talking to the nurses and arranging that phones would be easily accessible for both Ray and Rebecca so they could talk to each other. With help from cooperative nurses, Ray and Rebecca became roommates sharing the same hospital room. They both found comfort being together.

Cardiovascular Disease Includes Heart Attack, Stroke and Congestive Heart Failure

Cardiovascular disease (CVD) includes both the heart and blood vessels of the human body. Heart attack, stroke and congestive heart failure are three life-threatening, life-altering cardiovascular conditions discussed in this chapter.

According to a 2011 American Heart Association update, cardiovascular disease caused death to more than 251.2 per 100,000 Americans during 2007. Heart disease is ranked first as the cause of death for men and women. A demographic breakdown of those deaths reveals the rate of death among white men was 294 per 100,000 while deaths among white women number 205 per 100,000. Black males died at a rate or 405 per 100,000 while black women died at a rate of 286 per 100,000. During the decade of 1997–2007, the death rate declined 27.8 percent. However, these statistics still show an average of one death every 39 seconds.[1]

Many women worry about cancer but the facts show that coronary heart disease kills more women annually than the next two threats to their lives (breast cancer and lung cancer): "In the United States in 2007, all cardiovascular diseases combined claimed the lives of 421,918 females while all forms of cancer combined to kill 270,018. Breast cancer claimed the lives of 40,599 females; lung cancer claimed 70,388."[2] That means that over 10 times as many women die of heart disease as succumb to breast cancer.

Symptoms of a Heart Attack and What Causes Those Symptoms

Symptoms of a heart attack may include chest discomfort, pressure, squeezing or pain. This discomfort may also be experienced in one or both arms, the upper back, the jaw, the neck or the stomach. Shortness of breath may be a symptom of heart attack. Other symptoms include fatigue, sweating, and feeling nauseated or dizzy. Women may experience the same symptoms as men. However, doctors are recognizing that women often have subtle symptoms such as fatigue, being short of breath and feeling nauseated. In the past, women have often not taken their symptoms seriously and have not gotten help when they need it. The American Heart Association wants women to remember that heart and vascular disease is the number one killer of American women.[3]

What is a heart attack and what happens during a heart attack? A heart attack (myocardial infarction) occurs when the blood supply to the heart muscle is compromised. Not only does the inside of the heart pump blood, but the heart muscle itself must also have a blood supply to function properly. The coronary arteries carry oxygenated blood to the heart muscle. If the inside of those coronary arteries are clogged with plaque, the heart muscle cannot get enough blood and oxygen and a heart attack occurs. A combination of factors may cause this situation. One of the major causes involves atherosclerosis (hardening of the arteries).

Atherosclerosis means the inside layer of arteries have plaque attached to them. This plaque decreases the size of the artery and can cause blood clots when the blood flow past the plaque becomes sluggish. High cholesterol levels contribute to atherosclerosis, with its increased risk of heart attack and stroke. Approximately 37 million Americans have high cholesterol levels (240 mg/dL or greater).[4]

A diagnosis of a heart attack begins with a patient telling of recent symptoms and continues with a 12-lead electrocardiogram. This is a noninvasive test for which it takes only a few minutes to obtain the results. Electrodes are attached to the chest, arms and legs and the electrical activity of the heart is recorded onto paper. Doctors and nurses will compare the results to a normal EKG. Ischemia (inadequate blood and oxygen supply) of the heart muscle can often be detected by EKG changes. Doctors also look for arrhythmias (abnormal rhythm changes) when looking at EKGs.

Blood tests may be drawn to rule out or confirm a heart attack and may include Troponin T, creatine kinase and myoglobin. A variety of tests may be done to confirm that a heart attack has occurred or is likely to occur. These include stress tests, echocardiograms, nuclear cardiac imaging tests, cardiac MRI and CT tests, cardiac catheterization and angiograms. An exercise stress test involves a person walking on a treadmill while he is monitored by medical personnel. This person is watched for signs and symptoms of a heart attack. His blood pressure and EKG are monitored. If a person cannot walk on the treadmill because of other conditions, "pharmacologic" or IV medications can be used to stress the heart and identify a pending heart attack. Nuclear cardiac imaging tests involve injecting a radioactive solution such as Thallium, and a gamma camera is used to tell the doctor the status of the blood supply to the heart muscle and whether damage from a heart attack has occurred. Cardiac MRI and CT scans also evaluate the heart function and whether the blood supply to the heart muscle is healthy or compromised.

Treatments for Heart Attack

Cardiac catheterization and angiogram have become common in patients whose blood supply to their heart muscle is being evaluated. During a cardiac catheterization procedure, special catheters are inserted into a large vein (often in the groin area) and slid up the inside of the vein into the heart. During the angiogram portion, fluoroscopic X-ray views are taken, and contrast dye may be injected and films obtained which show whether a blockage exists. During this procedure, doctors may do tests to learn whether the heart muscle is healthy or damaged from a heart attack. During this procedure, a stent may be inserted into the coronary artery to improve blood flow. Balloon angioplasty may be done. During balloon angioplasty, a special balloon is slid up into the heart through a vein and inflated for a specific length of time, thus compressing the plaque and allowing improved blood flow. For some patients, this procedure will provide adequate help. For other patients, these tests will show that coronary bypass graft surgery is needed.

Coronary bypass graft surgery involves harvesting a piece of blood vessel from the patient (often a vein from the lower leg) and suturing the piece to the heart. This new blood vessel will carry an adequate blood supply past the blocked area and thus provide a blood supply to the heart muscle.

Symptoms of a Stroke and What Happens

Symptoms of a stroke include "sudden numbness or weakness of the face, arm or leg, especially on one side of the body, sudden confusion, trouble speaking or understanding, sudden trouble seeing in one or both eyes, sudden trouble walking, dizziness, loss of balance or coordination, sudden severe headache with no known cause."[5]

A person is displaying symptoms listed above and might be having a stroke. Ask him to smile. (Does he smile by moving both sides of his face evenly and with ease?) Ask him to close his eyes and raise both arms. (Does he understand and move both arms upward with ease and keep them up?) Ask him to repeat a simple sentence. (Does he understand and is his speech understandable?) If he shows problems with these tasks, call 911 immediately for help.[6]

A stroke occurs when the blood supply to an area of the brain is blocked by plaque or a blood clot (called ischemic stroke) or the blood vessel ruptures and bleeds into brain tissue (called hemorrhagic stroke). Symptoms occur because the brain tissue isn't getting the blood supply and oxygen it needs.

Diagnosis and Treatment for Stroke

Diagnosis of a stroke begins with recent history—what symptoms happened, time frame and current illnesses. Imaging studies such as MRI and CT scans may be done and physicians will use these studies to identify the type of stroke (ischemic or hemorrhagic) and appropriate treatment. A patient with ischemic stroke probably needs the tissue plasminogen activator (tPA) clot-busting treatment, while the person with hemorrhagic stroke does not need tPA.

A person experiencing stroke symptoms needs emergency medical care. Call 911 for emergency services and get medical treatment immediately. If the stroke is caused by a blockage in the blood supply, the first three hours of symptoms are the appropriate time for clot-busting drugs such as tPA to be given. When given within the three-hour time frame, tPA has been proven to decrease the damage done by a stroke. In a hemorrhagic stroke, the symptoms are caused by a ruptured blood vessel with bleeding around brain tissue. This type of stroke may require emergency surgery (craniotomy) to control bleeding and remove excess blood.

"Post stroke treatment is aimed at preventing recurrent stroke and medical complications, while promoting the fullest possible recovery of function."[7] Rehabilitation of stroke victims begins quickly. With the help of doctors, nurses and therapists, a stroke victim and his family learn exercises, both mental and physical, in their efforts to regain their prior level of functioning.

Symptoms of Congestive Heart Failure (CHF) and What Happens

"In the United States, **5.8** million people have heart failure. One in five people die within one year of diagnosis."[8] Congestive heart failure is present when the pumping efforts of a person's heart are inadequate. This inefficient pumping by the heart means less blood is ejected out of the heart each time it contracts and inadequate blood flow and oxygen go to body organs. The blood volume may become backed up and leak out at the capillaries of the body, which results in shortness of breath and swollen tissues, especially of the feet and legs. The symptoms of CHF include being short of breath, wheezing and having difficulty breathing — especially when lying down — fatigue, limited ability to exercise, having swollen feet, lower legs and abdomen, being cyanotic (blueness or duskiness) — especially fingernails and mucous membranes such as the lips — heart palpitations, and confusion during acute episodes.

Seventy-four percent of Americans who develop CHF have high blood pressure (above 140/90). Damage to the heart muscle during a heart attack and high blood cholesterol levels contribute to development of CHF. Doctors who talk to their patients about their high blood pressure readings are trying to prevent CHF, strokes and heart attacks.[9]

Diagnosis and Treatment for Congestive Heart Failure

A person's doctor will consider several possible causes for congestive heart failure when making a diagnosis. While talking with the patient and the family, doctors will want to know about symptoms such as shortness of breath, a cough, feeling fatigued, etc. The physician may order laboratory tests or an electrocardiogram which will identify any heart rhythm problems. An echocardiogram will tell the doctors more about heart function. A chest X-ray may show an enlargement of the heart. Cardiac MRI and CT scan may also be done. For an acute life-threatening episode of congestive heart failure, more invasive monitoring might be needed.

Treatment for congestive heart failure aims to improve the pumping efficiency of the heart. There's no cure for congestive heart failure, but management of symptoms can improve a person's life and help prevent more damage. Diuretics (water pills) help get rid of excess fluid within the body. A cardiologist may tell a person to eat less salt (salt contributes to fluid retention and overload within the blood vessel system). Prescription heart medications such as digitalis help to strengthen the heart muscle's contraction and efficiency. For persons with end-stage heart failure, mechanical assistance machines and heart transplantation may be needed.

Important Structures and How They Function

"The heart is a four-chambered muscular pump approximately the size of a man's fist that beats an average of 70 times each minute, 24 hours a day, 365 days each year for a lifetime. In 1 day, this pump moves more than 1800 gallons of blood throughout the body, and the work performed by the heart over a lifetime would lift 30 tons to a height of 30,000 feet."[10]

The heart's four chambers are named the right atrium, the right ventricle, the left atrium and the left ventricle. The right and left atriums serve as collection reservoirs. The right atrium collects oxygen-poor blood returning from the body to the heart. When the right-side valve called the tricuspid valve opens, the blood flows from the atrium into the ventricle. The valve shuts behind it and prevents the blood from backing up into the atrium. The right ventricle contracts and the blood inside is forced into the pulmonary artery, which carries the deoxygenated blood into the lungs.

Inside the pulmonary circulation (inside the lung) the carbon dioxide is removed from the blood and oxygen is added to the blood. Then the oxygen-rich blood is returned to the left atrium. The left-side valve between the atrium and ventricle is called the bicuspid valve. This valve opens, the blood flows from the atrium into the ventricle and this valve closes. With the next contraction of the ventricle, the oxygenated blood is pushed out into the aorta (the largest artery of the body) and travels up to the brain and out to the rest of the body (except the lungs) via arteries.

The lungs function in the oxygenation of blood and removal of carbon dioxide as the blood travels through the pulmonary circulation system. This gas-exchange activity occurs in the tiny alveoli of the lungs. With each breath a person takes, the lungs take oxygen out of the air and add this oxygen to the blood. The carbon dioxide which the lungs take out of the blood is exhaled with every breath.

Arteries carry oxygenated blood from the heart to body tissues. The largest artery is called the aorta, which attaches to the left side of the heart. The aorta branches off into smaller arteries that attach to even smaller arteries called arterioles, and arterioles attach to tiny capillaries. Capillaries are the tiny blood vessels. Body tissues obtain nutrition and oxygen and give up waste materials and carbon dioxide at the capillaries. "In each person, there are approximately 10 billion capillaries, with a total surface area of 500 to 700 m^2."[11]

Veins carry deoxygenated blood from the body back to the heart. The smallest veins called venules, collect the blood containing waste materials and carbon dioxide from the capillaries and return it to the larger veins, which join together and become the vena cava, the body's largest vein. The vena cava attaches to the right atrium. This cycle of blood flow never stops until a person dies.

Blood is the liquid found in the body's circulatory system. It's made up of yellow serum, red blood cells, white blood cells, and platelets: "Blood accounts for about 7% to 8% of total body weight. The total volume of blood in the average adult is about 5 to 6 L (liters), and it circulates throughout the body within the confines of the circulatory system."[12]

Blood cells include red blood cells (called erythrocytes.) Red blood cells carry oxygen using a protein called hemoglobin (HgB). White blood cells (WBCs) are called leukocytes. WBCs keep a person's immune system strong by fighting off infections, identifying and destroying cancer cells, and assisting in the inflammatory response and wound healing. Three major types of WBCs include granulocytes, lymphocytes and monocytes.

The granulocytes are divided into three subtypes called neutrophils, eosinophils and basophils. Neutrophils protect the body from bacteria, fungi, and foreign substances when they secrete enzymes to harm the invader. Eosinophils are involved in allergic reactions and fighting off parasite infections. Basophils are involved with allergic reactions. The lymphocytes, often identified by names such as B cells, T cells, and natural killer cells, defend a body from microorganisms. Lymphocytes secrete deadly chemicals called cytokines and antibodies to protect the body. Monocytes could be likened to "Pac-Man" because they are scavengers, swallowing up harmful foreign material. "They digest the dead enemy and remove injured tissue."[13] They also play a role in chronic inflammation and activate other WBCs such as lymphocytes.

What causes the heart to contract and pump blood? An electrical system built into the heart causes the routine contraction. The electrical signal begins in the "pacemaker" area of the heart called the SA (sinoatrial) node and follows its pathway across the atrium and ventricle. The signal causes both the atrium and the ventricle to contract and then rest/recover before the next electrical impulse occurs. This electrical activity of the heart is recorded on the electrocardiogram (EKG) tracing. Problems in the electrical system of the heart can cause problems. For example, atrial fibrillation occurs when an abnormal heart rhythm causes inefficient emptying of the blood from the atria into the ventricles. Small blood clots can form and travel to the brain, causing a stroke, or to the coronary arteries, causing a heart attack.

Prevention Strategies for Cardiovascular Disease

Risk factors increase a person's chance of heart attack and cardiovascular disease. Some of those risk factors, such as age, sex and genetic makeup, cannot be changed. However, a person can change behaviors that put him at increased risk, such as beginning to exercise, avoiding smoking and drinking too much alcohol, managing stress or eating too much unhealthy food. Other risk factors include high blood pressure, high blood cholesterol, being overweight, and uncontrolled diabetes. Each person should talk to his doctor for an individualized plan for preventing heart and cardiovascular disease.

Go for a walk or a swim. Exercise helps prevent cardiovascular disease. A 30-minute activity 5 days a week meets the recommendation by the American Heart Association. Exercise helps in many ways: it decreases stress level, lowers blood pressure, lowers the blood levels of LDL while increasing the blood levels of HDL and helps keep weight at a healthy level. For people who struggle to get a 30-minute time frame to exercise, doing three 10-minute exercises is a good alternative. Taking 10 minutes of the lunch hour to walk about the work place may be a good exercise break.

Stop smoking. "Cigarette smoking is the most important preventable cause of premature death in the United States." As many as 440,000 American smokers die every year.[14] People searching for help in quitting smoking can find it at http://www.smokefree.gov/.

Drink alcohol in moderation. The recommended amount is one drink for women and two drinks for a man per day. The experts believe this amount of alcohol puts a person at lower risk of CVD than no alcohol intake. However, drinking more than the recommended amount puts a person at risk of high blood pressure and high triglycerides and can contribute to cancer, obesity, alcoholism, accidents and suicide.

Eat healthy food. "Your skin, which has covered you since your birth, is replaced entirely by new cells every seven years. The fat beneath your skin is not the same fat that was there a year ago. Your oldest red blood cell is only 120 days old, and the entire lining of your digestive tract is renewed every 3 to 5 days. To maintain your 'self,' you must continually replenish, from foods, the energy and nutrients you deplete as your body maintains itself."[15] Food is more than, say, a cheeseburger and fries. Food becomes your body cells. What goes into your mouth is changed into building blocks which your body uses to repair, rebuild and replenish itself. The AHA recommended healthy diet includes fresh fruits and vegetables, whole-grain and high-fiber foods, lean meat and fish and low-fat dairy products.

Lower high blood pressure. Blood pressure measures the pressure inside blood vessels when the heart pumps (the top number called systolic) and when the heart rests (the bottom number called diastolic). When those numbers are elevated, it's called high blood pressure or hypertension. If high blood pressure isn't treated and brought down to normal levels, damage can occur to the heart, blood vessels, and organs, such as the kidneys.

A normal blood pressure for adults is a systolic below 120 mm Hg and a diastolic below 80mm Hg (120/80). A slight elevation in blood pressure (120–139/80–89) would be monitored by a person's doctor. If and when the numbers become routinely higher, treatment will be considered. Lower blood pressure can sometimes be achieved by lifestyle changes. See chapter 10 for more information about high blood pressure.

Avoid high blood cholesterol. What is cholesterol? Why is LDL called bad cholesterol and HDL called good cholesterol? What does a cholesterol level of 250 mean? Triglycerides and cholesterol are two lipids (fats) needed by the human body. Fats have gotten a reputation for causing heart disease but they are necessary. Fats (triglycerides) provide fuel and are necessary for healthy cell structure. Cholesterol is utilized by the body when it makes hormones, bile and vitamin D. More details on cholesterol and lipid profile results can be found in chapter 10.

The three major components of food are categorized as carbohydrates, proteins and fats. While fats are crucial parts of nutrition, they have 9 calories (nutritionists say 9 kilocalorie/gram of fat compared to 4 kilocalorie/gram of carbohydrate or protein). The goal is to eat healthy fats in small amounts daily and use up (by exercising) the same number of calories taken in by eating and drinking. When a person eats more food than he uses up in exercise output, the body converts the excess to adipose (fat) and stores it.

Maintain a health weight. Worldwide, over 1.7 billion people are overweight. In the United States, more than 65 percent of adults are overweight or obese. "Obesity results from an imbalance between energy intake and energy consumption. Because fat is the main storage form of energy, obesity represents an excess of body fat."[16] It sounds easy: move more and eat less. But many people struggle with their weight. Suggested strategies include eating more fruits and vegetables, substituting water for sugared beverages, increasing activity, decreasing the amount of time spent at non-active pastimes such as watching television or being on a computer.[17]

Control diabetes. Diabetes increases the risk of cardiovascular disease. Sixty-five percent of people with diabetes die with heart and blood vessel disease. More information about diabetes can be found in chapter 14.

Keep teeth and gums healthy. Does gum disease increase a person's risk of heart disease? Experts looked at 120 studies and concluded that gum disease puts a person at increased risk for heart attack and blood vessel disease because of the infection and inflammation around the teeth and gums. See chapter 10 for prevention and treatment of gum disease.

Research

Cardiovascular disease affects many people, and ongoing research into prevention and the best treatments continue. Over 8000 studies, past and present, can be found at the National Institutes of Health Website (www.clinicaltrials.gov) when the words "heart disease" are typed into the search function.

Smoking increases a person's risk of death due to heart disease and cancer. Adults numbering 12,152 were included in a study which found that smokers face a 2.58 times increased risk of death from all causes and a 2.26 times increased risk from heart disease.[18]

"More hospitals are administering emergency stroke drug, but many patients don't seek treatment quickly enough to get it." This study, reported in 2009, showed that only 37 percent of stroke patients arrived at the hospital within two hours of the onset of stroke symptoms (so tests could be done and the tPA, or clot-busting drug, could be given within the three-hour time frame). The researchers found that people with more severe symptoms were more than twice as likely to arrive within the recommended time frame. They also noted that black patients were 44 percent less likely to arrive at the hospital within the two-hour recommended time frame. A new recommendation (2009) from the American Heart Association/American Stroke Association recommends that tPA be given up to 4.5 hours after symptoms begin for certain patients.[19]

High blood cholesterol contributes to congestive heart failure. Researchers looked at the blood cholesterol levels of 6860 men and women in the Framingham Heart Study over a period of 26 years. They found that 13 percent of those with elevated LDL and triglycerides developed congestive heart failure compared with only 7.9 percent of those with normal levels of LDL. The researchers were surprised when they found that only 6 percent of those with high HDL levels developed congestive heart failure while 12 percent who had a low HDL developed congestive heart failure. They concluded that "this study goes a step further in implicating cholesterol levels (both HDL and LDL) in heart failure and suggests that cholesterol-altering therapy may have long-term benefits in preventing heart failure above and beyond its effects on preventing myocardial infarction."[20]

Being overweight or obese and not exercising contributed to heart failure. The Physicians Health Study followed 21,094 American male doctors age 40 to 84 for 20 years. Compared to lean, active participants, the risk of heart failure increased 19 percent in the lean and inactive, 49 percent in the active, overweight men; 78 percent in the inactive, overweight men; 168 percent in the active, obese men, and 293 percent in the inactive, obese men. Among the doctors involved in this study, exercise activity levels ranged from one to three times a month to daily exercise. Any amount of aerobic exercise which resulted in sweating was considered beneficial.[21]

When compared to a woman who did not walk for exercise, a woman who walks for 2 or more hours a week has a 30 percent decreased risk of suffering any type of stroke. This research included over 39,000 healthy American women age 45 and older who participated in the Women's Healthy Study for over 11 years. These researchers found that walking as exercise decreased a woman's risk of all types of stroke, including ischemic and hemorrhagic.[22]

Caregivers and the Disease

Three common heart and cardiovascular events which affect both caregivers and their family members are heart attacks, stroke and congestive heart failure. When a person experiences a heart attack or stroke, family members rally around and cheer their loved one. Some people will be fortunate enough to recover completely without any loss of function. Others will find their stamina gone and their ability to use an arm and a leg (often on the same side) is impaired. Rebecca found her weakened heart condition could not be cured but could be managed with her doctor's help.

During the adjustment time after medical crisis, many emotions will surface. The person dealing with a recent heart attack or stroke may find himself very afraid — of another event. Loving family members may find themselves trying too hard, not sure whether to do everything for the person recovering from a stroke or whether to watch him struggle as he tries to eat, spilling food off the spoon. The recommended behavior is to encourage the person to work toward independence and recovery. When recovery ends, gently help him accept his reality, which may mean facing limitations. Many people experience depression after a heart attack, heart surgery or a stroke. Caregivers should discuss this situation with the person's doctors for help and guidance.

Caregivers helping people with heart conditions must recognize that caregiving may be needed for a long time. The caregivers must pace themselves, put their own needs as a top priority, and plan for relaxing time away from their caregiving responsibilities, taking time to exercise, relax and reward self with peaceful solitude. Caregivers must communicate with family, friends and co-caregivers to get the best for self and their loved ones.

Glossary

Activities of daily living (ADLs) behaviors such as bathing, dressing and self-care activities which an individual needs to be able to perform to care for self.

Acupuncture the use of fine needles inserted at specific points on the skin. Acupuncture is primarily used for pain relief.

Acute pain short-term pain suffered due to an injury. Short-term pain goes away when the body heals from the injury.

Adverse reaction an unwanted effect caused by the administration of drugs. Onset may be sudden or develop over time. (See side effects.)

Benign not cancer, or non malignant.

Bone spurs small growths of bone that can occur on the edges of a joint affected by osteoarthritis. These bone spurs are also called osteophytes.

Cancer an abnormal cell mass that grows uncontrollably. It may spread (metastasize) to other parts of the body. Cancer is one word that refers to over 100 different diseases. Doctors may refer to cancer as malignancy, malignant tumor or malignant neoplasm.

Cartilage a hard, slippery coating on the end of bones. The breakdown of this cartilage is a part of osteoarthritis.

Catecholamines chemicals the body makes and releases in times of stress and the "fight or flight" response. These chemicals include epinephrine, norepinephrine and dopamine. These chemicals are also available for medical use.

Cholesterol a necessary form of fat which the human body uses to make bile, hormones and energy metabolism.

Chondrocytes components of cartilage. Chondrocytes are cells that produce cartilage and are found throughout cartilage and help it stay healthy as it grows. Chondrocytes can release enzymes that destroy collagen and other proteins.

Chronic pain pain that lasts past the time of healing.

Collagen a family of fibrous proteins that are components of cartilage. Collagens are the building blocks of skin, tendon, bone and other connective tissues.

Complementary and Alternative therapy a broad range of healing philosophies, approaches and therapies that Western (conventional) medicine does not commonly use to promote well-being or to treat health conditions.

Congestive heart failure (CHF) a condition in which the heart pumps inefficiently, whether from a rhythm problem or a weakened heart muscle

Contraindication a specific circumstance when the use of certain treatments could be harmful.

Corticosteroids powerful anti-inflammatory hormones that are made naturally in the body or are man-made for use as medicine. Corticosteroids may be injected into the affected joints to temporarily reduce inflammation and relieve pain.

Diabetes mellitus a condition in which the blood sugar level is abnormally high.

Diabetic ketoacidosis a potentially life-threatening condition in which the blood sugar levels are too high while the body cells break down fats to get energy. Ketones result from the breakdown of fat. High levels of ketone and blood sugar occur, resulting in diabetic ketoacidosis, which most commonly affects persons with type 1 diabetes, not type 2.

DNA (deoxyribose nucleic acid) one of the molecules which contains genetic information.

Durable power of attorney for healthcare a legal document used by an individual who designates one to make decisions about the individual's medical care if he is unable to make them.

Frostbite ice crystals formed within soft tissues due to being exposed to cold.

General anesthesia a level of anesthesia where a person is unconscious of what happens around him

Gingivitis inflammation and infection of the gum tissue around teeth.

Glucosamine a substance that occurs naturally in the body and provides the building blocks to make and repair cartilage.

Heat exhaustion a condition where a person loses large amounts of fluids and salt through sweating and becomes dehydrated and ill.

Heat stroke when one overheats to dangerous levels because he is past heat exhaustion.

High density lipoprotein (HDL) "good" cholesterol.

Hospice a medical service used to provide physical, emotional and spiritual care to a person and his family when a cure isn't possible.

Hyaluronic acid a substance that gives healthy joint fluid its slippery property. Hyaluronic acid may be reduced inside osteoarthritic joints. Replacing the hyaluronic acid (with Viscosupplement injections) may reduce pain, increase lubrication and improve function for some people.
Hyperosmolar hyperglycemic State (HHS) a life-threatening occurrence brought about when the blood sugar goes high and serious dehydration occurs. A person with type 2 diabetes may have an HHS crisis.
Hypertension higher-than-normal blood pressure.
Hypoglycemia when blood sugar is abnormally low and if untreated can become a life-threatening situation. People with both type 1 and type 2 diabetes can have a hypoglycemic episode.
Hypothermia abnormally cold body temperature.
In situ within the normal area. An in situ tumor has not spread outside the area of the body it was found in.
Instrumental activities of daily living (IADL) include meal preparation, clothing care, and home maintenance activities.
Islets of Langerhans area of the pancreas where insulin is produced.
Joint capsule a tough membrane that holds the bones and joint parts together.
Living will a legal document which spells out what medical care (life-prolonging measures) an individual wants if he is unable to speak or make the decision.
Low-density lipoprotein (LDL) "bad" cholesterol.
Magnetic resonance imaging (MRI) provides high resolution computerized images of internal body tissues. The machine uses a strong magnet that passes a force through the body to create the images.
Metastasis cancer cells that have spread from one part of the body to another.
Mitochondria powerhouse of the cell.
Myocardial infarction a condition where the blood supply to a portion of the heart is blocked and tissue of that area of the heart may die—another name for heart attack.
Neoplasm a tumor or abnormal new grouping of cells. The word is often used to mean cancer but not always. One should ask the doctor whether he means cancer or a benign tumor.
Nonsteroidal anti-inflammatory drugs (NSAIDs) a class of medicines available over the counter or with a prescription to ease pain and inflammation. Commonly used NSAIDS include ibuprofen (Motrin, Advil), naproxen sodium (Aleve) and ketoprofen (Oorudis, oruvail).
Nucleus (of a cell) control center of the cell.
Osteoarthritis the most common form of arthritis. It is known as the cause of the breakdown of joint cartilage, resulting in pain, stiffness and disability.
Osteophytes small growths of bone that appear on the edges of a joint affected by osteoarthritis, also known as bone spurs.

Periodontal disease advanced infection and inflammation of gums and teeth.

Polypharmacy (many drugs) problems, side effects, or interactions caused by taking several drugs, whether prescription, over-the-counter or herbal and vitamin supplements.

Power of attorney a legal document used when an individual designates someone to handle business affairs when the individual is unable to do so.

Prognosis expected outcome. A doctor may predict a patient's expected outcome based on the patient's health status.

Proteoglycans components of cartilage. Made up or proteins and sugars, strands of proteoglycans interweave with collagens and form a mesh-like tissue. This allows cartilage to flex and absorb physical shock.

Regional anesthesia anesthesia where nerve sensation is blocked to a specific area of the body and for a specific time. Spinal anesthesia is an example.

Respite temporary relief for a caregiver when someone takes over the care of the loved one and gives the caregiver a break or vacation.

Side effects any undesired actions or effects of a drug or treatment. Negative or adverse side effects may include a variety of problems, including headache, nausea, hair loss, skin irritation and other physical problems.

Stroke, or cerebrovascular accident (CVA) occurs when the blood supply to an area of the brain is blocked (called an ischemic stroke) or a blood vessel ruptures and bleeds into brain tissue (called a hemorrhagic stroke).

Synovial fluid a fluid secreted by the synovium that lubricates the joint and keeps the cartilage smooth and healthy.

Synovium a thin membrane inside the joint capsule that secretes synovial fluid.

Telomere the end of a chromosome where DNA replicates itself.

Triglycerides a measurement in a cholesterol panel test. Triglyceride level reflects a person's genetics and excess food eaten and not utilized.

Tumor an abnormal mass or group of cells. A tumor can be cancerous or benign (not cancer).

X-ray a procedure in which low-level radiation is passed through the body to produce a picture called a radiograph. X-rays of joints affected by osteoarthritis can show such things as cartilage loss, bone damage and bone spurs.

Chapter Notes

Chapter 1

1. U.S. Department of Health and Human Services, "Health, United States, 2007," www.cdc.gov/nchs/data/hus/hus07.pdf#027.
2. Centers for Disease Control (CDC), "Ten Great Public Health Achievements — United States, 1900–1999," http://cdc.gov/mmwr/preview/mmwrhtml/00056796.htm.
3. Census Reports, Twelfth Census of the United States taken in 1900, http://www.cdc.gov/nchs/data/vsushistorical/vsush_1900_3.pdf.
4. Centers for Disease Control (CDC), "Deaths: Final Data for 2005," http://www.cdc.gov/nchs/data/nvsr/nvsr56/nvsr56_10.pdf.
5. U.S. Department of Health and Human Services, "A Statistical Profile of Older Americans Aged 65+," www.h-gac.com/human-services/aging/documents/AStatisticalProfileofOlderAmericansAged65plus.pdf.
6. National Family Caregivers Association, "Caregiving Statistics," www.nfcacares.org/who_are_family_caregivers/care_giving_statistics.cfm.
7. *Ibid.*
8. *Ibid.*
9. Area Agency on Aging of Pasco-Pinellas, "Are you a Caregiver?" www.agingcarefl.org/caregiver/caregiver.
10. C. Goldman, *The Gifts of Caregiving, Stories of Hardship, Hope and Healing* (Minneapolis, Fairview, 2002), 7, 69.
11. National Family Caregivers Association, "Caregiving Statistics," www.nfcacares.org/who_are_family_caregivers/care_giving_statistics.cfm.
12. *Ibid.*
13. Pasco-Pinellas County Florida Area Agency on Aging, "Four Stages of Caregiving," http://www.agingcarefl.org/caregiver/fourstages.
14. USAA Education Foundation, "Effects of Aging on Driving Skills," www.usaaedfoundation.org/DownloadRelatedForm/535_Recent_Driving_Experiences_Checklist.pdf.
15. Beth Witrogen McLeod, *Caregiving* (New York: John Wiley& Sons, 1999), 20–21.
16. Pasco-Pinellas County Florida Area Agency on Aging, "Four Stages of Caregiving," http://www.agingcarefl.org/caregiver/fourstages.
17. Caregiver Resource Center, Corporate Services, http://www.caregiverresourcecenter.com/corporate_services.htm.

18. U.S. Department of Labor, Employment Standards Administration, Family and Medical Leave Act, http://www.dol.gov/whd/fmla/finalrule/factsheet.pdf.
19. CDC, "Falls Among Older Adults: An Overview," http://www.cdc.gov/HomeandRecreationalSafety/Falls/adultfalls.html.
20. Pasco-Pinellas County Florida Area Agency on Aging, "Four Stages of Caregiving," http://www.agingcarefl.org/caregiver/fourstages.
21. MayoClinic.com, "Forgiveness: How to Let Go of Grudges and Bitterness," http://www.mayoclinic.com/health/forgiveness/MH00131/.
22. *Ibid.*
23. *Ibid.*

Chapter 2

1. Cindy Brotherton, personal interview with the author, June 1, 2010.
2. Childstats.gov, "America's Children: Key National Indicators of Well-being, 2009 Highlights," http://childstats.gov/pdf/ac2009/ac_09.pdf.
3. Cindy Brotherton, personal interview with the author, June 1, 2010.
4. Elisabeth Kubler-Ross & David Kessler, The Five Stages of Grief, http://grief.com/the-five-stages-of-grief/.
5. J.W. Worden, *Grief Counseling and Grief Therapy: A Handbook for the Mental Health Practitioner*, 3rd ed. (New York: Springer, 2002).
6. *Ibid.*, 29.
7. *Ibid.*, 30.
8. *Ibid.*, 34.
9. *Ibid.*, 37.
10. Cindy Brotherton, personal interview with the author, June 1, 2010.
11. *Ibid.*
12. *Ibid.*
13. M.J. Hockenberry, *Wong's Essentials of Pediatric Nursing* (St. Louis: Elsevier Mosby, 2005), 556
14. *Ibid.*, 556.
15. Cindy Brotherton, personal interview with the author, June 1, 2010.
16. *Ibid.*
17. *Ibid.*
18. National Alliance for Caregiving, "Young Caregivers in the U.S.," http://www.caregiving.org/data/youngcaregivers.pdf.
19. *Ibid.*
20. L. Austin, "Children as Caregivers, Today's Caregiver," http://www.caregiver.com/articles/children/children_as_caregivers.htm.
21. University of Iowa Health Science Relations, "Children and Critically Ill Parents: What Children Need to Know," http://www.uihealthcare.com/topics/medicaldepartments/pediatrics/childrenillparents/index.html.
22. Austin, "Children as Caregivers," http://www.caregiver.com/articles/children/children_as_caregivers.htm.
23. Worden, *Grief Counseling*, 160.
24. *Ibid.*, 160–161.
25. *Ibid.*, 163.
26. *Ibid.*, 161.
27. Hockenberry, *Wong's Essentials*, 556.
28. *Ibid.*, 556.
29. *Ibid.*, 87.
30. *Ibid.*, 88.
31. *Ibid.*
32. *Ibid.*
33. *Ibid.*

Chapter 3

1. Beth W. McLeod, *Caregiving: The Spiritual Journey of Love, Loss and Renewal* (New York: John Wiley & Sons,1999) 3.
2. Family Caregiver Alliance, Fact Sheet: "Taking Care of YOU: Self-Care for Family Caregivers," http://www.caregiver.org/caregiver/jsp/content_node.jsp?nodeid=847).
3. American Heart Association (AHA), "Reality Check," http://www.americanheart.biz/HEARTORG/Caregiver/RealityCheck/RealityCheckIntroduction/Reality-Check-Introduction_UCM_301769_Article.jsp.
4. National Family Caregivers Association, "Caregiving Statistics," http://www.nfcacares.org/who_are_family_caregivers/care_giving_statstics.cfm.
5. National Institute of Mental Health, "Research Shows How Chronic Stress May Be Linked to Physical and Mental Ailments," http://www.nimh.nih.gov/science-news/2009/research-shows-how-chronic-stress-may-be-linked-to-physical-and-mental-ailments.shtml.
6. National Institutes of Health (NIH), "Stressed Out?" http://newsinhealth.nih.gov/pdf/NIHNiHJanuary07.pdf.
7. National Family Caregiver, "Caregivers and Your Health: How to Manage Stress," http://nfcacares.org/pdfs/Evercare_caregiver_stress.pdf.
8. MayoClinic.com, "Healthy Lifestyles," http://www.mayoclinic.com/health/HealthyLivingIndex/HealthyLivingIndex.
9. American Cancer Society, "Diet and Physical Activity: What's the Cancer Connection?" http://www.cancer.org/cancer/CancerCauses/DietandPhysicalActivity/diet-and-physicalactivity.
10. National Family Caregivers Association, "The Best Present You Can Give Your Loved One: Your Own Good Health," http://www.nfcacares.org/pdfs/ProtectYourHealth.pdf.
11. U.S. Department of Health and Human Services, Administration of Aging, "Be Wise — Immunize," http://www.caregiver.org/caregiver/jsp/content/pdfs/English_final1.2.pdf.
12. NIH News in Health, "Stressed Out?" http://newsinhealth.nih.gov/pdf/NIHNiHJanuary07.pdf.
13. American Heart Association, "Reality Check," http://www.americanheart.biz/HEARTORG/Caregiver/RealityCheck/RealityCheckIntroduction/Reality-Check-Introduction_UCM_301769_Article.jsp.
14. McLeod, *Caregiving* (New York: John Wiley & Sons,1999) 14.
15. National Family Caregivers Association, "Caregiving Statistics," http://www.nfcacares.org/who_are_family_caregivers/care_giving_statstics.cfm).
16. National Family Caregivers Association, "The Stress of Family Caregiving," http://nfcacares.org/pdfs/TakeCareWinter06.pdf.
17. Freedom from Fear, "An Overview of Depression," http://www.freedomfromfear.org/depressionoverview.asp.
18. "Fight-or-Flight Versus Tend-and-Befriend: The Significance of Gender Differences in Stress Responses," http://obssr.od.nih.gov/pdf/taylor_slides.pdf.
19. David Niven, *The 100 Simple Secrets of Healthy People* (New York: HarperSanFrancisco, 2003) 136.
20. "Prayer and Spirituality in Health: Ancient Practices, Modern Science," www.jpsych.com/pdfs/NCCAM-PrayerandSpirituality.pdf.
21. Sue Wessel, personal interview with the author, September 2010.
22. "Prayer and Spirituality in Health," www.jpsych.com/pdfs/NCCAM-PrayerandSpirituality.pdf.
23. WebMD, "Caregivers Tip No. 1: Take Care of Yourself First," http://www.webmd.com/balance/tc/caregiver-tips-caregiver-tip-number-1-take-care-of-yourself-first.
24. WebMD, "Caregiver Burnout," http://women.webmd.com/caregiver-recognizing-burnout.
25. "Children of Aging Parents: Strategies for Avoiding Burnout During Caregiving," http://www.caps4caregivers.org/Assets/CAPSsummer2007B.pdf.

26. National Sleep Foundation, "Can't Sleep? What to know about insomnia," http://www.sleepfoundation.org/article/sleep-related-problems/insomnia-and-sleep.
27. National Sleep Foundation, "One-Third of Americans Lose Sleep Over Economy," http://www.sleepfoundation.org/article/press-release/one-third-americans-lose-sleep-over-economy.
28. H. Delehanty and E. Ginzler, *Caring for Your Parents: The Complete Family Guide* (New York: Sterling, 2005), 165.
29. Science Daily, "Comfort-food Cravings May Be Body's Attempt to Put Brake on Chronic Stress," http://www.sciencedaily.com/releases/2003/09/030911072109.htm.
30. Family Caregivers Online, Module 9, "Caring for the Caregiver," www.familycaregiversonline.com/family_caregiver_module.asp?module=17.
31. American Heart Association, "Rejuvenate," http://www.heart.org/HEARTORG/Caregiver/Rejuvenate/RejuvenateIntroduction/Rejuvenate-Introduction_UCM_301816_Article.jsp.
32. Ibid.
33. Health and Age, "Exercise Helps Caregivers Manage Stress," http://www.healthandage.org/Exercise-Aids-Stressed-Caregivers.
34. Niven, *100 Simple Secrets*, 147.
35. Ibid., 148.
36. Ibid., 99.
37. Ibid., 173.
38. Niven, *100 Simple Secrets of the Best Half of Life* (San Francisco: HarperCollins, 2005), 120.
39. B. Jacobs, *The Emotional Survival Guide for Caregivers* (New York: Guilford, 2006), 62.
40. Ibid., 63.
41. AARP, "How to Deal with Long-Distance Issues," http://www.aarp.org/relationships/caregiving-resource-center/info-09-2010/pc_tips_for_long_distance_caregiver.html.
42. Ibid.
43. Family Caregiver Alliance, "Siblings and Caregiving," http://www.caregiver.org/caregiver/jsp/content_node.jsp?nodeid=653.

Chapter 4

1. Brainy Quotes, "Voltaire," http://brainyquote.com/quotes/keywords/longer.html.
2. H. Delehanty and E. Ginzler, *Caring for your Parents: The Complete Family Guide* (New York: Sterling, 2005), 162.
3. J. Horstman, *The Arthritis Foundation's Guide to Alternative Therapies* (Atlanta: Arthritis Foundation, 1999), 78.
4. D. Niven, *The 100 Simple Secrets of Healthy People* (New York: Harper Collins, 2003), 52.
5. Ibid.
6. Horstman, *Guide to Alternative Therapies*, 79.
7. Ibid., 83.
8. W. Robiner, "Psychological and Physical Reactions to Whirlpool Baths," *Journal of Behavioral Medicine* 13, no. 2 (1990), 157–173, http://www.springerlink.com/content/r100363044650082/.
9. American Heart Association, "Reality Check," http://www.americanheart.biz/HEARTORG/Caregiver/RealityCheck/RealityCheckIntroduction/Reality-Check-Introduction_UCM_301769_Article.jsp.
10. *Arthritis Today Walking Guide*, "The Perfect Fit," 7.
11. Ibid.
12. Robert S. Dinsmoore, "Taking Up Walking One Step at a Time," *Arthritis Self-Management* 6, no. 5, 17–23.

13. American Massage Therapy Association (AMTA) "Massage and Serious Health Conditions," http://www.amtamassage.org/findamassage/health_conditions.html.
14. American Massage Therapy Association (AMTA), "Massage Therapy Can Relieve Stress," http://www.amtamassage.org/statement2.html.
15. Horstman, *Guide to Alternative Therapies*, 122.
16. ATMA, "Choosing a Type of Massage," www.amtamassage.org/findamassage/massage_type.html.
17. E. Zimney, "Gardening Is Good Exercise," http://www.everydayhealth.com/blog/zimney-health-and-medical-news-you-can-use/gardening-is-good-exercise/.
18. Centers for Disease Control, "Be Healthy and Safe in the Garden," http://cdc.gov/features/gardeningtips.
19. Horstman, *Guide to Alternative Therapies*, 109.
20. *Ibid.*, 110.
21. S. Crotzer, "Yoga for Arthritis," *Arthritis Self-Management* (Sept/Oct 2004), 23–28.
22. WebMD.com, "His and Hers Stress Advice," http://women.webmd.com/features/stress-tips-for-men-and-women.
23. A. Klein, *The Courage to Laugh* (New York: Penguin Putnam, 1998), 10.
24. Holistic Online, "Therapeutic Benefits of Laughter," http://www.holisticonline.com/Humor_Therapy/humor_therapy_benefits.htm.
25. Klein, *Courage*, 4.
26. Niven, *100 Simple Secrets*, 99.
27. Klein, *Courage*, 26.
28. B.J. Jacobs, *The Emotional Survival Guide for Caregivers* (New York: Guildford, 2006)137.
29. Niven, *100 Simple Secrets*, 126.
30. D. Niven, *100 Simple Secrets of the Best Half of Life* (San Francisco: HarperCollins, 2005), 131.
31. M. Ramos, "Music Therapy," Mindmovers," http://www.mindmovers.com/store/music.htm.
32. National Institutes of Health, "Can Pets Help Keep You Healthy?" http://newsinhealth.nih.gov/2009/February/feature1.htm.
33. Centers for Disease Control, "Health Benefits of Pets," http://www.cdc.gov/healthypets/health_benefits.htm.
34. Health Journeys, "What Is Guided Imagery?" www.healthjourneys.com/what_is_guided_imagery.asp.
35. Horstman, *Guide to Alternative Therapies*, 62.
36. *Ibid.*, 91.
37. A. Klein, *The Simplify-Your-Life Quote Book* (New York: Random House, 2005), 37.
38. B.J. Jacobs, *The Emotional Survival Guide for Caregivers* (New York: Guildford Press, 2006), 86.
39. Think Exist Quotes.com, "Buddha Quote," http://thinkexist.com/quotes/buddha/3.html.

Chapter 5

1. National Family Caregivers Association, "21st Century Caregiving — Then and Now," http://www.thefamilycaregiver.org/who_are_family_caregivers/then_and_now.cfm.
2. E.K. Abel, *Hearts of Wisdom: American Women Caring for Kin* (Cambridge: Harvard University Press, 2000), 263.
3. *Ibid.*, 37–38.
4. *Ibid.*, 75.
5. Ira Rutlow, *Seeking the Cure: A History of Medicine in America* (New York: Scriber, 2010), 46.

6. John C. Gunn, *Gunn's Domestic Medicine* (Knoxville: University of Tennessee Press, 1986), 440. This edition is a reprint of the originally published *Gunn's Domestic Medicine, or, Poor Man's Friend,* "Printed under the immediate superintendence of the author, a physician of Knoxville, 1830."
7. U.S. Department of Health and Human Services, "Health, United States, 2007," http://www.cdc.gov/nchs/data/hus/hus07.pdf#027.
8. Development for Professional Employees, "Professional Women: Vital Statistics Fact Sheet, 2006," http://www.pay-equity.org/PDFs/ProfWomen.pdf.
9. Rutlow, *Seeking the Cure,* 17.
10. *Ibid.*, 10.
11. Centers for Disease Control and Prevention, "Smallpox Disease Overview," http://www.bt.cdc.gov/agent/smallpox/overview/disease-facts.asp.
12. "Zabdiel Boylston and Inoculation," http://www.todayinsci.com/B/Boylston_Zabdiel/Boylston_Zabdiel.htm.
13. Rutlow, *Seeking the Cure,* 16.
14. *Ibid.*, 37.
15. *Ibid.*, 39.
16. *Ibid.*, 125.
17. *Ibid.*, 153.
18. "History of Medicine Timeline," http://www.history-timelines.org.uk/events-timelines/10-history-of-medicine-timeline.htm.
19. P.G. Barash, B.F. Cullen, and R.K. Stoelting, *Clinical Anesthesia* (Philadelphia: J.B. Lippincott, 1989), 3.
20. *Ibid.*, 7.
21. *Ibid.*, 11.
22. *Ibid.*, 13.
23. S.E. Hohler, *Arthritis: A Patient's Guide* (Jefferson, NC: McFarland, 2008) 39.
24. University of Dayton, "History of the Microscope," http://campus.udayton.edu/~hume/Microscope/microscope.htm.
25. "Louis Pasteur," http://www.historylearningsite.co.uk/louis_pasteur.htm.
26. "Lister and Antisepsis, 1867–1967," *American Journal of Public Health* 57 (1967):1899–1900, http://ajph.aphapublications.org/cgi/reprint/57/11/1899.
27. D. Humphreys, "Historic Operating Room: A Monument to the Advent of Antisepsis," *Canadian Medical Association Journal* 178, no. 2 (January 15, 2008): 93–194, http://www.ncbi.nlm.nih.gov/pmc/articles/PMC2175006/.
28. *Ibid.*
29. "Fleming, Alexander," *New World Encyclopedia,* http://www.newworldencyclopedia.org/entry/Alexander_Fleming.
30. Rutlow, *Seeking the Cure,* 23.
31. E.K. Abel, *Hearts of Wisdom: American Women Caring for Kin* (Cambridge: Harvard University Press, 2000), 69.
32. *Ibid.*, 40.
33. J. Harlow, "Eight Decades of Health Care, Hospitals and Health Networks," http://www.hhnmag.com/hhnmag_app/jsp/articledisplay.jsp?dcrpath=HHNMAG/Article/data/03MAR2007/0703HHN_FEA_80Anniv&domain=HHNMAG.
34. American Hospital Association, "Fact Facts on US Hospitals," http://www.aha.org/aha/resource-center/Statistics-and-Studies/fast-facts.html.
35. V.L. Holder, "From Handmaiden to Right Hand: The Infancy of Nursing," *AORN Journal* 79, no. 2, 374–390.
36. *Ibid.*, 448–464.
37. B.G. Ulmer, "Army Nurse Corps Celebrates 100th Anniversary," *AORN Journal* 73, no. 1, 8–12.
38. Unitarian Universalist Historical Society, "Clara Barton," http://www25.uua.org/uuhs/duub/articles/clarabarton.html.
39. Holder, "From Handmaiden to Right Hand," 618–632.
40. *Ibid.*, 448–464.

41. D.J. Brooks, "Rating the Ethics of Medical Professionals," http://www.gallup.com/poll/7417/Rating-Ethics_Medical_Professionals.aspx.
42. Michigan State University, "Alzheimer's Disease Timeline," http://hod.kcms.msu.edu/timeline.php?y=all.
43. P.A. Dervan, *Understanding Cancer* (Jefferson, NC: McFarland, 1999), 11.
44. American Cancer Society, "The History of Cancer," http://www.cancer.org/docroot/CRI/content/CRI_2_6x_the_history_of_cancer_72.asp.

Chapter 6

1. G. Kanegan and M. Boyette, *How to Survive Your Hospital Stay* (New York: Simon & Schuster, 2003), 62.
2. Centers for Medicare and Medicaid, "Medicare and You," http://www.medicare.gov/Publications/Pubs/pdf/10050.pdf.
3. David Sherer and M. Karinch, *Dr. David Sherer's Hospital Survival Guide: 100+ ways to Make Your Hospital Stay Safe and Comfortable* (Washington, DC: Claren, 2003), 10.
4. Family Doctor.org, "Tips for Talking to Your Doctor," http://familydoctor.org/online/famdocen/home/pat-advocacy/healthcare/837.html.
5. Kanegan and Boyette, *How to Survive Your Hospital Stay*, 18.
6. Sherer and Karinch, *Dr. David Sherer's Hospital Survival Guide*, 223.
7. S.E. Hohler, *Arthritis: A Patient's Guide* (Jefferson, NC: McFarland, 2008), 139.
8. American Occupational Therapy Association Fact Sheet, "Home Modifications and Occupational Therapy," http://www.aota.org/Practitioners/PracticeAreas/Rehab/Tools/385 11.aspx.
9. B.J. Jacobs, *The Emotional Survival Guide for Caregivers* (New York: Guilford, 2006), 39–40.
10. Kanegan and Boyette, *How to Survive Your Hospital Stay*, 10.
11. Hohler, *Arthritis*, 138.
12. M.F. Roizen, M.C. Oz and The Joint Commission, *You, the Smart Patient: An Insider's Handbook for Getting the Best Treatment* (New York: Free Press, 2006), 86.
13. Hohler, *Arthritis*, 140.
14. Roizen, Oz and The Joint Commission, *You the Smart Patient*, 267.
15. *Ibid.*, 275.
16. Medicare.gov, "Medicare Advantage Part C," http://www.medicare.gov/navigation/medicare-basics/medicare-benefits/part-c.aspx.
17. Hospice, "The Hospice Concept," http://www.hospicenet.org/html/concept.html.
18. Centers for Medicare and Medicaid Services, Medicare Hospice Benefits, http://www.medicare.gov/Publications/Pubs/pdf/02154.pdf.
19. P.A. Dervan, *Understanding Cancer* (Jefferson, NC: McFarland, 1999), 7.
20. Roizen, Oz and The Joint Commission, *You the Smart Patient*, 124.
21. University of Chicago, "Polypharmacy in Older Adults," http://prescriptions.uchicago.edu/Polypharmacy/symptoms.html.
22. American Geriatrics Society, Foundation for Health in Aging, "Avoid Overmedication and Harmful Drug Reactions," http://www.healthinaging.org/public_education/avoiding_overmedication.pdf.
23. Kanegan and Boyette, *How to Survive Your Hospital Stay*, 115.
24. American Academy of Family Doctors, "Antibiotics: When They Can and Can't Help," http://familydoctor.org/online/famdocen/home/common/infections/protect/680.html.
25. *Ibid.*
26. C.P. Adams and V.V. Brantner, "Estimating The Cost of New Drug Development: Is It Really $802 Million?" *Health Affairs* 25, no.2 (2006): 420–428, http://content.healthaffairs.org/cgi/content/full/25/2/420.

Chapter 7

1. U.S. Department of Health and Human Services, Centers for Disease Control and Prevention, "National Health Statistics Reports," July 30, 2008, http://www.cdc.gov/nchs/data/nhsr/nhsr005.pdf.
2. *Merck Manual of Health and Aging,* "Undergoing Surgery," http://www.merckmanuals.com/home/special_subjects/surgery/surgery.html.
3. D. Sherer and M. Karinch, *Dr. David Sherer's Hospital Survival Guide* (Washington: Claren, 2003), 18–21.
4. University of Maryland Medical Center, Robotic Surgery Program, http://www.umm.edu/robotics/faq.htm.
5. Caregivers Library, "Infection Control," http://www.caregiverslibrary.org/Default.aspx?tabid=481.
6. Center for the Advancement of Health (November 20, 1999), "Depression Alters Immune Systems by Depressing Physical Activity," *ScienceDaily,* http://www.sciencedaily.com/releases/1999/11/991130062958.htm.
7. Ashar Ata, J. Lee, S. Bestle, J. Desemone and S. Stain, "Postoperative Hyperglycemia and Surgical Site Infection in General Surgery Patients," *Archives of Surgery* 145, no. 9 (September 2010), http://archsurg.ama-assn.org/cgi/content/short/145/9/858.
8. C.M. Porth and G. Matfin, *Pathophysiology: Concepts of Altered Health States,* 8th ed. (Philadelphia: Wolters Kluwer Health/Lippincott Williams & Wilkins, 2009), 354.
9. The Joint Commission, "Five Things You Can Do to Prevent Infection," Speak UP initiative, http://www.jointcommission.org/Speak_Up_Five_Things_You_Can_Do_To_Prevent_Infection/.
10. Centers for Disease Control and Prevention, "Wash Your Hands," http://www.cdc.gov/Features/HandWashing/.
11. Porth and Matfin, *Pathophysiology,* 1603.
12. *Ibid.,* 757, 1604.
13. "Prothrombin Time (PT)," Medline Plus, http://www.nlm.nih.gov/medlineplus/ency/article/003652.htm.
14. Heart Rhythm Society, "INR," http://www.heartrhythmfoundation.org/a-fib/INR_FINAL.pdf.
15. "Partial Thromboplastin Time (PTT)," Medline Plus, http://www.nlm.nih.gov/medlineplus/ency/article/003653.htm.
16. S.E. Hohler, *Arthritis: A Patient's Guide* (Jefferson, NC: McFarland, 2008),186.
17. *Ibid.,* 189.

Chapter 8

1. American Bar Association, *You and Your Aging Parents* (New York: Random House, 2009), 34–35.
2. Jessica Hill, personal interview with the author, 11/2010.
3. Full Circle of Care Caregiver Website, "Activities of Daily Living," http://www.fullcirclecare.org/ltcontinuum/everydaytasks.html.
4. H. Delehanty E. Ginzler, *Caring for Your Parents* (New York: Sterling, 2005), 142.
5. C.M. Porth and G. Matfin, *Pathophysiology: Concepts of Altered Health States* (Philadelphia: Wolters Klower Health/Lippincott Williams & Wilkins, 2009), 47.
6. Laurence Z. Rubenstein, "Falls in Older People: Epidemiology, Risk Factors and Strategies for Prevention," *Age and Ageing* (2006), 35–52, http://ageing.oxfordjournals.org/content/35/suppl_2/ii37.full.pdf.
7. AGS Foundation for Health in Aging, "Preventing Serious Falls: Tips for Older Adults and Their Loved Ones," http://www.healthinaging.org/public_education/falls_tips.pdf.

8. Rubenstein, "Falls in Older People," 35–52, http://ageing.oxfordjournals.org/content/35/suppl_2/ii37.full.pdf.
9. American Geriatrics Society, Foundation for Health in Aging, "Winter Safety Tips for Older Adults," http://www.healthinaging.org/public_education/wintersafety_tips.pdf.
10. *Ibid.*
11. InterNACHI, "Home Safety for the Elderly," http://www.nachi.org/elderlysafety.hml.
12. *Ibid.*
13. American Geriatrics Society, Foundation for Health in Aging, "Winter Safety Tips for Older Adults," http://www.healthinaging.org/public_education/wintersafety_tips.pdf.
14. Administration on Aging, "Heat Illnesses and Tips for Preventing Illness During Hot Weather," http://www.aoa.gov/AoARoot/Preparedness/Resources_Individuals/Heat_Illness.aspx.
15. WebMD, "Understanding Heat-Related Illness — Treatment," http://firstaid.webmd.com/understanding-heat-related-illness-treatment.
16. American Geriatrics Society, Foundation for Health in Aging, "Winter Safety Tips for Older Adults."
17. WebMD, "Hypothermia Treatment," http://firstaid.webmd.com/hypothermia-treatment.
18. American Geriatrics Society, Foundation for Health in Aging, "Winter Safety Tips for Older Adults," http://www.healthinaging.org/public_education/wintersafety_tips.php.
19. WebMD, "Frostbite Treatment," http://firstaid.webmd.com/frostbite-treatment.
20. American Geriatrics Society, Foundation for Health in Aging, "Emergency Preparedness Tips for Older Adults," http://www.healthinaging.org/public_education/emergency_tips.php.
21. *Ibid.*
22. American Bar Association, *You and Your Aging Parents* (New York: Random House, 2009), 247.

Chapter 9

1. Peggy Gross, personal interview with the author, February 7, 2011.
2. *Ibid.*
3. Greg Gross, permission to include eulogy, February 12, 2011.
4. Michael Gross, permission to include eulogy, February 21, 2011.
5. Gregory (Keith) Gross, permission to include eulogy, February 15, 2011.
6. Peggy Gross, personal interview with the author, February 7, 2011.
7. M. Colgrove, H.H. Bloomfield and P. McWilliams, *How to Survive the Loss of a Love* (Los Angeles: Prelude, 1991), a.
8. J.W. Worden, *Grief Counseling and Grief Therapy* (New York: Springer, 2002), 7–8.
9. *Ibid.*, 9.
10. *Ibid.*, 12–15.
11. *Ibid.*, 12
12. *Ibid.*, 13.
13. *Ibid.*, 23
14. *Ibid.*, 27.
15. *Ibid.*, 30.
16. *Ibid.*, 32.
17. Peggy Gross, personal interview with the author, February 7, 2011.
18. Worden, *Grief Counseling*, 35.
19. Colgrove, Bloomfield and McWilliams, *How to Survive the Loss of a Love*, 36.
20. J.R. White, *Grieving: Our Path Back to Peace* (Minneapolis: Bethany House, 1997), 84.
21. Worden, *Grief Counseling*, 137.
22. Peggy Gross, personal interview with the author, February 7, 2011.

23. Worden, *Grief Counseling*, 140.
24. Peggy Gross, personal interview with the author, February 7, 2011.
25. Worden, *Grief Counseling*, 140.
26. *Ibid.*, 125.
27. B.J. Jacobs, *The Emotional Survival Guide for Caregivers* (New York: Guilford, 2006), 20.
28. WebMD, "Mental Health and Adjustment Disorder," http://www.webmd.com/mental-health/mental-health-adjustment-disorder.
29. Jacobs, *The Emotional Survival Guide*, 21.
30. Peggy Gross, personal interview with the author, February 7, 2011.
31. *Ibid.*
32. Colgrove, Bloomfield and McWilliams, *How to Survive the Loss of a Love*, 42.
33. *Ibid.*, 72.
34. *Ibid.*, 106.
35. *Ibid.*, 122.
36. A. Klein, *The Courage to Laugh* (New York: Penguin Putnam, 1998), 194.
37. *Ibid.*, 187.
38. B. Poor and G.P. Poirrier, *End of Life Nursing Care* (Sudbury, MA: Jones and Bartlett, 2001), 48.
39. Peggy Gross, personal interview with the author, February 7, 2011.

Chapter 10

1. M.F. Roizen and M.C. Oz, *You Staying Young: The Owner's Manual for Extending Your Warranty* (New York: Simon & Schuster, 2007) 12.
2. "Nurses Health Study," *Nurses' Health Study Annual Newsletter* 14 (2007), http://www.channing.harvard.edu/nhs/wp-content/uploads/n2007.pdf.
3. Roizen and Oz, *You Staying Young*, 41.
4. Harvard School of Public Health press release, "Active Social Life May Delay Memory Loss among U.S. Elderly Population," http://www.hsph.harvard.edu/news/press-releases/2008-releases/active-social-life-delay-memory-loss-us-elderly.html.
5. "Nurses Health Study."
6. King's College, "Exercise in Leisure Time Prolongs Life," http://www.kcl.ac.uk/news/news_details.php?year=2008&news_id=729.
7. E.S. Epel, E.H. Blackburn, J. Lin, F.S. Dhabhar, N.E. Adler, J.D. Morrow and R.M. Cawthon, "Accelerated Telomere Shortening in Response to Life Stress," http://www.ncbi.nlm.nih.gov/pmc/articles/PMC534658/.
8. S.E. Hohler, *Arthritis: A Patient's Guide* (Jefferson, NC: McFarland, 2008), 96.
9. *Science Daily*, "Walking Associated with Lower Stroke Risk in Women," http://sciencedaily.com/releases/2010/04/1000406162945.htm.
10. C.M. Porth and G. Matfin, *Pathophysiology: Concepts of Altered Health States* (Philadelphia: Wolters Klower Health/Lippincott Williams & Wilkins, 2009), 512.
11. *Ibid.*, 514.
12. National Heart, Lung and Blood Institute, "Your Guide to Lowering Blood Pressure," http://www.nhlbi.nih.gov/health/public/heart/hbp/hbp_low/hbp_low.pdf.
13. Porth and Matfin, *Pathophysiology*, 482.
14. "Nurses Health Study."
15. *Ibid.*
16. Roizen and Oz, *You Staying Young*, 64.
17. National Center for Health Statistics, "Overweight Prevalence Among Adults, 2005–2006," http://www.cdc.gov/nchs/data/hestat/overweight/overweight_adult.htm.
18. Rand Corporation, "Why People Overeat," http://www.rand.org/pubs/research_briefs/RB9327/index1.html.
19. "Nurses Health Study."

20. National Institute of Neurological Disorders, "Brain Basics: Understanding Sleep," http://www.ninds.nih.gov/disorders/brain_basics/understanding_sleep.htm.
21. National Institutes of Health, "Sleep Apnea Tied to Increased Risk of Stroke," http://www.nih.gov/news/health/apr2010/nhlbi-08.htm.
22. American Sleep Apnea Association, *Tired of the Sleepiness?*, http://www.sleepapnea.org/resources/brochure.html.
23. American Sleep Apnea Association, "Treatment Options for Adults with Obstructive Sleep Apnea," http://www.sleepapnea.org/resources/pubs/treatment.html.
24. R. Berent, J. Auer, P. Schmid, G. Krannmair, S.F. Crouse and J.S. Green, "Periodontal and Coronary Heart Disease in Patients Undergoing Coronary Angiography," *Metabolism* 60, no. 1 (2011): 127–133, http://www.ncbi.nlm.nih.gov/pubmed/20096894.
25. American Dental Association, "Preventing Periodontal Disease," *Journal of American Dental Association* 132 (September 2001), http://www.ada.org/sections/ScienceAndResearch/pdfs/patient_08.pdf.
26. M.S. Tonetti, F. D'Aiuto, L. Nibali, A. Donald, C. Storrey, M. Parkar, J. Suvan, A. Hingorani, P. Vallance and J. Deanfield, "Treatment of Periodontitis and Endothelial Function," *New England Journal of Medicine* 356, 911–920, http://www.nejm.org/doi/full/10.1056/NEJMoa063186.
27. CBS News, "Bad Habits Can Age You by 12 Years Study Shows," http://www.cbsnews.com/stories/2010/04/26/health/main6434223.shtml.
28. E. Kvaavik, D. Batty, G. Ursin, R. Huxley and C. Gale, "Influence of Individual and Combined Health Behaviors on Total and Cause-Specific Mortality in Men and Women," *Archives of Internal Medicine* 170: 8, http://archinte.ama-assn.org/cgi/content/short/170/8/711.

Chapter 11

1. Alzheimer's Association, "What is Alzheimer's?," http://www.alz.org/alzheimers_disease_what_is_alzheimers.asp.
2. P.B. Smith, M.M. Kenan and M.E. Kunik, *Alzheimer's for Dummies* (Hoboken, NJ: Wiley, 2004), 9.
3. *Ibid.*, 24.
4. National Institutes of Health, "Alzheimer's Disease Genetics Fact Sheet," http://www.nia.nih.gov/Alzheimers/Publications/geneticsfs.htm.
5. Alzheimer's Association, "Brain Tour," http://www.alz.org/alzheimers_disease_4719.asp.
6. M.F. Roizen and M.C. Oz, *You Staying Young: The Owner's Manual for Extending Your Warranty* (New York: Simon & Schuster, 2007), 43.
7. Alzheimer's Society, "Mediterranean Diet Decreases Dementia," International Conference on Alzheimer's Disease 2009, http://www.alzheimers.org.uk/site/scripts/news_article.php?newsID=506.
8. Roizen and Oz, *You Staying Young*, 31.
9. Mayo Clinic, "Diabetes and Alzheimer's Linked," http://www.mayoclinic/health/diabetes-and-alzheimers/AZ00050.
10. International Conference on Alzheimer's Disease (ICAD), 2009 Press Release, http://www.alzheimers.org.uk/site/scripts/news_article.php?newsID=499.
11. Alzheimer's Society, "Physical Activity Can Prevent Grey Matter Shrinkage," http://www.alzheimers.org.uk/site/scripts/news_article.php?newsID=814
12. R.S. Wilson, K.R. Krueger, S.E. Arnold, J.A. Schneider, J.F. Kelly, L.L. Barnes et al., "Loneliness and Risk of Alzheimer's Disease," *Archives of General Psychiatry* 64, no. 2 (2007): 234–240. http://archpsyc.ama-assn.org/cgi/content/abstract/64/2/234.
13. C.B. Hall, R.B. Lipton, M. Sliwinski, M.J. Katz, C.A. Derby and J. Verghes, "Cognitive Activities Delay Onset of Memory Decline in Persons Who Develop Dementia," *Neurology* 73 (2009): 356–361, http://www.neurology.org/cgi/content/abstract/73/5/356.

14. S. Halpern, *Can't Remember What I Forgot* (New York: Harmony, 2008), 4–5.
15. Alzheimer's Association, "10 Warning Signs of Alzheimer's Disease," http://www.alz.org/alzheimers_disease_10_signs_of_alzheimers.asp.
16. C.M. Porth and G. Matfin, *Pathophysiology: Concepts of Altered Health States* (Philadelphia: Wolters Klower Health/Lippincott Williams & Wilkins, 2009), 1210–11.
17. Smith, Kenan and Kunik, *Alzheimer's for Dummies*, 10.
18. Alzheimer's Association, "Brain Tour," http://www.alz.org/brain/08.asp.
19. Smith, Kenan and Kunik, *Alzheimer's for Dummies*, 47.
20. "Neurological History and Examination," http://www.patient.co.uk/doctor/Neurological-History-and-Examination.htm.
21. Alzheimer's Association, Alzheimer's Association, "Steps to Diagnosis," http://www.alz.org/alzheimers_disease_steps_to_diagnosis.asp.
22. Alzheimer's Association, "Ten Signs of Alzheimers," http://www.alz.org/alzheimers_disease_10_signs_of_alzheimers.asp.
23. Alzheimer's Association, "Standard Treatments," http://www.alz.org/alzheimers_disease_standard_prescriptions.asp.
24. University of Pennsylvania School of Medicine, "Targeting Tau: Inflammation Study Suggests New Approach for Fighting Alzheimer's," http://www.uphs.upenn.edu/news/News_Releases/jan07/microglia-activation-alzheimers.htm.
25. Alzheimer's Association, "Dressing and Grooming," http://alz.org/living_with_alzheimers_dressing_and_grooming.asp.
26. Alzheimer's Research Foundation, "10 Trips for Traveling with Your Loved One," http://www.alzinfo.org/06/articles/caregiving-52.
27. Research in Review, "A Book for the Mind," http://www.rinr.fsu.edu/fallwinter9899/features/book.html.

Chapter 12

1. J.H. Klippel, *Primer on the Rheumatic Diseases* (Atlanta: Arthritis Foundation, 2001), 286.
2. S.E. Hohler, *Arthritis: A Patient's Guide* (Jefferson, NC: McFarland, 2008), 4.
3. Klippel, *Primer*, 285.
4. Arthritis Foundation, "Osteoarthritis Fact Sheet," http://www.arthritis.org/media/newsroom/osteoarthritis_Fact_Sheet_from_AF-Find_12_10_09.pdf.
5. *Ibid.*
6. Klippel, *Primer*, 287.
7 Hohler, *Arthritis*, 7
8. C.M. Porth, G. Matfin, *Pathophysiology: Concepts of Altered Health States* (Philadelphia: Wolters Klower Health/Lippincott Williams & Wilkins, 2009), 1535.
9. National Institute of Arthritis and Musculoskeletal and Skin Diseases, "Osteoarthritis," http://www.niams.nih.gov/Health_Info/Osteoarthritis/default.asp#2.
10. *Ibid.*
11. Kate Lorig and James Fries, *The Arthritis Helpbook*, 5th ed. (Cambridge: Perseus, 2000), 122.
12. American Academy of Orthopaedic Surgeons (AAOS), "Viscosupplement Treatment for Arthritis," http://www.orthoinfo.aaos.org/topic.cfm?topic=a00217.
13. National Center for Complementary and Alternative Medicine (NCCAM), "Acupuncture Relieves Pain and Improves Function in Knee Osteoarthritis," http://nccam.nih.gov/research/results/spotlight/052504.htm.
14. D. Foltz-Gray, *Alternative Treatments for Arthritis* (Atlanta: Arthritis Foundation, 2005), 41.
15. *Ibid.*, 42.
16. Hohler, *Arthritis*, 129.

17. American Massage Therapy, "Massage Therapy Industry Fact Sheet, 2009," http://www.amtamassage.org/research/Consumer-Survey-Fact-Sheets/2009-Consumer-Survey-Fact-Sheet.html.
18. Foltz-Gray, *Alternative Treatments*, 162.
19. Intelihealth, "Meditation," http://www.intelihealth.com/IH/ihtIH?d=dmtContent&c=362173&p=~br,IHW~st,24479~r,WSIHW000×~b,*.
20. Foltz-Gray, *Alternative Treatments*,163.
21. National Institutes of Health News Advisory; National Center for Complementary and Alternative Medicine, National Institutes of Health, "More Than One-Third of U.S. Adults Use Complementary and Alternative Medicine, According to New Government Survey," http://nccam.nih.gov/news/2004/052704.htm.
22. Gallup News Service, "Who Believes in God and Who Doesn't?," June 23, 2006, http://www.gallup.com/poll/23470/Who-Believes-God-Who-Doesnt.aspx.
23. Gallup News Service, "Very Religious Americans Lead Healthier Lives," December 23, 2010, http://www.gallup.com/poll/145379/Religious-Americans-Lead-Healthier-Lives.aspx.
24. Arthritis Today, "5 Steps to Pain Relief," http://www.arthritistoday.org/treatments/self-treatments/5-steps-to-pain-relief-2.php.
25. *Hypography Science for Everyone*, "High Heels Bad News for Knees," http://hypography.com/news/life-sciences/30688.html.
26. Arthritis Foundation, "Clarifying the Role of Fat in Osteoarthritis," http://www.arthritis.org/role-of-fat-in-osteoarthritis.php.
27. NCCAM, "Dietary Supplements Glucosamine and/or Chondroitin Fare No Better Than Placebo in Slowing Structural Damage of Knee Osteoarthritis," http://nccam.nih.gov/news/2008/092908.htm.

Chapter 13

1. C. Kip Bennett, personal interview with the author, 2/4/2010.
2. *Ibid.*
3. C.M. Porth and G. Matfin, *Pathophysiology: Concepts of Altered Health States*, 8th ed. (Philadelphia: Wolters Kluwer Health/Lippincott Williams & Wilkins, 2009), 156.
4. American Cancer Society, "Cancer Facts and Figures, 2010," http://www.cancer.org/acs/groups/content/@epidemiologysurveilance/documents/document/acspc-026238.pdf.
5. American Cancer Society, "Signs and Symptoms of Cancer," http://www.cancer.org/Cancer/CancerBasics/signs-and-symptoms-of-cancer.
6. Porth and Matfin, *Pathophysiology*, 57.
7. Peter A. Dervan, *Understanding Cancer: A Scientific and Clinical Guide for the Layperson* (Jefferson, NC: McFarland, 1999), 26.
8. American Cancer Society, "Guidelines for the Early Detection of Cancer," http://www.cancer.org/Healthy/FindCancerEarly/CancerScreeningGuidelines/american-cancer-society-guidelines-for-the-early-detection-of-cancer.
9. R. Mishori, "Stay Healthy: Do Alternative Cancer Therapies Work?," *Parade*, December 6, 2009, pg. 18.
10. American Cancer Society, "What in Cigarette Smoke Is Harmful?," http://www.cancer.org/Cancer/CancerCauses/TobaccoCancer/QuestionsaboutSmokingTobaccoandHealth/questions-about-smoking-tobacco-and-health-cancer-and-health.
11. American Cancer Society, "Diet and Physical Activity: What's the Cancer Connection?," http://www.cancer.org/Cancer/CancerCauses/DietandPhysicalActivity/diet-and-physical-activity.
12. American Cancer Society, "How Do I Protect Myself from UV?," http://www.cancer.org/Cancer/CancerCauses/SunandUVExposure/SkinCancerPreventionandEarlyDetection/skin-cancer-prevention-and-early-detection-u-v-protection.
13. *Ibid.*
14. *Ibid.*

15. C. Kip Bennett, personal interview with the author, 2/4/2010.
16. *Ibid.*

Chapter 14

1. Jan Gile, personal interview with the author, 9/15/2010.
2. Sue Wessel, personal interview with the author, 9/15/2010.
3. Centers for Disease Control (CDC), "National Diabetes Fact Sheet, 2007," http://www.cdc.gov/diabetes/pubs/pdf/ndfs_2007.pdf.
4. *Ibid.*
5. C.M. Porth and G. Matfin, *Pathophysiology: Concepts of Altered Health States*, 8th ed. (Philadelphia, PA: Wolters Kluwer Health/Lippincott Williams & Wilkins, 2009), 1049.
6. *Ibid.*, 1053.
7. *Ibid.*, 1051.
8. S.R. Rolfes, K. Pinna and E. Whitney, *Understanding Normal and Clinical Nutrition*, 8th ed. (Belmont CA: Wadsworth, 2009), 9.
9. Porth and Matfin, *Pathophysiology*, 1055.
10. American Diabetes Association, "Checking Your Blood Glucose," http://www.diabetes.org/living-with-diabetes/treatment-and-care/blood-glucose-control/checking-your-blood-glucose.html.
11. U.S. Department of Health and Human Services, National Diabetes Education Program, "The Facts About Diabetes: America's Seventh Leading Cause of Death," http://ndep.nih.gov/diabetes-facts/index.aspx.
12. Centers for Disease Control, "National Diabetes Fact Sheet, 2007," http://www.cdc.gov/diabetes/pubs/pdf/ndfs_2007.pdf.
13. M.F. Roizen and M.C. Oz, *You Staying Young: The Owner's Manual for Extending Your Warranty* (New York: Simon & Schuster, 2007),149.
14. U.S. Department of Health and Human Services, NIH National Diabetes Education Program, "Get Real! You Don't Have to Knock Yourself Out to Prevent Diabetes," http://ndep.nih.gov/publications/PublicationDetail.aspx?PubId=76.
15. U.S. Department of Health and Human Services, National Diabetes Education Program, "Small Steps, Big Rewards: Your Game Plan to Prevent Type 2 Diabetes: Information for Patients," http://ndep.nih.gov/publications/PublicationDetail.aspx?PubId=71.
16. Centers for Disease Control, "National Diabetes Fact Sheet, 2007," http://www.cdc.gov/diabetes/pubs/pdf/ndfs_2007.pdf.
17. Katie Bond, personal interview with the author, 9/15/2010.
18. Centers for Disease Control, "National Diabetes Fact Sheet, 2007," http://www.cdc.gov/diabetes/pubs/pdf/ndfs_2007.pdf.
19. Porth and Matfin, *Pathophysiology*, 1047.
20. *Ibid.*, 1054.
21. Centers for Disease Control, "National Diabetes Fact Sheet, 2007," http://www.cdc.gov/diabetes/pubs/pdf/ndfs_2007.pdf.
22. Porth and Matfin, *Pathophysiology*, 1073.
23. Centers for Disease Control, "National Diabetes Fact Sheet, 2007," http://www.cdc.gov/diabetes/pubs/pdf/ndfs_2007.pdf.
24. *Ibid.*
25. *Ibid.*
26. Porth and Matfin, *Pathophysiology*, 1067.
27. Diabetes Research Institute, "Under the Microscope: Interview with Norma S. Kenyon, Ph.D.," http://www.diabetesresearch.org/Page.aspx?pid=1134.
28. National Institute of Diabetes and Digestive and Kidney Diseases, National Institutes of Health (NIH), "DCCT and EDIC: The Diabetes Control and Complications Trial and Follow-up Study," http://diabetes.niddk.nih.gov/dm/pubs/control/index.htm.
29. American Diabetes Association, "Diet, Exercise, Anti-diabetic Drugs Can Delay or

Prevent Type 2 Diabetes for 10+ Years," http://www.diabetes.org/news-research/research/recent/recent-advances/diet-exercise-anti-....

Chapter 15

1. American Heart Association, "Heart Disease and Stroke Statistics — 2011 Update," http://circ.ahajournals.org/content/123/4/e18.full.pdf.
2. American Heart Association, "Women and Cardiovascular Diseases, 2011 Update," http://heart.org/idc/groups/heart-public/@wcm/@sop/@smd/documents/downloadable/ucm_319576.pdf.
3. *Ibid.*
4. C.M. Porth and G. Matfin, *Pathophysiology: Concepts of Altered Health States* (Philadelphia, PA: Wolters Kluwer Health/Lippincott Williams & Wilkins, 2009), 480.
5. American Stroke Association, "Warning Signs," http://www.strokeassociation.org/STROKEORG/WarningSigns/Warning-Signs_UCM_308528_SUBHOMEPAGE.jsp.
6. National Stroke Foundation, "Warning Signs of Stroke," http://www.stroke.org/site/PageNavigator/ALS?Splash_20110907.html.
7. Porth and Matfin, *Pathophysiology,* 1324.
8. Centers for Disease Control, "Heart Failure Fact Sheet," http://cdc.gov/DHDSP/data_statistics/fact_sheets/fs_heart_failure.htm.
9. American Heart Association, "Why Blood Pressure Matters," http://www.heart.org/HEARTORG/Conditions/HighBloodPressure/WhyBloodPressureMatters/Why-Blood-Pressure-Matters_UCM_002051_Article.jsp.
10. Porth and Matfin, *Pathophysiology,* 457.
11. *Ibid.,* 471.
12. *Ibid.,* 254.
13. Peter A. Dervan, *Understanding Cancer: A Scientific and Clinical Guide for the Layperson* (Jefferson, NC: McFarland, 1999), 17.
14. American Heart Association, "Smoking and Cardiovascular Disease," http://www.heart.org/HEARTORG/GettingHealthy/QuitSmoking/QuittingResources/Smoking-Cardiovascular-Disease_UCM_305187_Article.jsp.
15. S.R. Rolfes, K. Pinna and E. Whitney, *Understanding Normal and Clinical Nutrition,* 8th ed. (Belmont CA: Wadsworth, 2009), 5.
16. Porth and Matfin, *Pathophysiology,* 993.
17. *Ibid.,* 995.
18. American Heart Association, "Smoking Remains Potent Risk Factor for Death from Heart Disease, Cancer," http://www.newsroom.heart.org/pr/aha/897.aspx.
19. American Heart Association, "More Hospitals Administering Emergency Stroke Drug, but Many Patients Don't Seek Treatment Quickly Enough to Get It," http://www.newsroom.heart.org/pr/aha/833.aspx.
20. American Heart Association, "Abnormal Cholesterol Levels May Raise Risk of Heart Attack," http://newsroom.heart.org/pr/aha/898.aspx.
21. *Medical News Today,* "Staying Lean and Fit Reduced Men's Risk of Heart Failure," http://medicalnewstoday.com/articles/134128.php.
22. *Science Daily,* "Walking Associated with Lower Stroke Risk in Women," http://www.medicalnewstoday.com/releases/2010/04/100406162945.htm.

Resources

Books

American Bar Association. *The American Bar Association Guide to Legal, Financial and Health Care Issues: You and Your Aging Parents*. New York: Random House Reference, 2009.
Delehanty, Hugh, and Elinor Ginzler. *Caring for Your Parents: The Complete Family Guide* (New York: AARP, 2005).
Foltz-Gray, Dorothy. *Alternative Treatments for Arthritis: An A to Z Guide to Herbs, Supplements, Bodywork and Other Complementary Treatments for Arthritis*, 2nd ed. (Atlanta: Arthritis Foundation, 2007).
Goldman, Connie. *The Gifts of Caregiving: Stories of Hardship, Hope and Healing* (Minneapolis: Fairview Press, 2002).
Hennessey, Maya. *If Only I'd Had This Caregiving Book* (Bloomington, IN: AuthorHouse, 2006).
Hohler, S.E. *Arthritis: A Patient's Guide* (Jefferson, NC: McFarland, 2008).
Jacobs, B.J. *The Emotional Survival Guide for Caregivers* (New York: Guilford Press, 2006).
Kanegan, G.V. *How to Survive Your Hospital Stay* (New York: Fireside, 2003).
Klein, Allen. *The Healing Power of Humor* (Los Angeles: Jeremy P. Tarcher, 1989).
Lorig, K., and J.F. Fries. *The Arthritis Helpbook*. 6th ed. (Cambridge: Da Capo, 2006).
McLeod, Beth Witrogen. *Caregiving: The Spiritual Journal of Love, Loss and Renewal* (New York: John Wiley, 1999).
Niven, David. *The 100 Simple Secrets of Healthy People* (New York: HarperCollins, 2003).
Roizen, M.F., and M.C. Oz. *You—The Smart Patient: An Insider's Handbook for Getting the Best Treatment* (New York: Free Press, 2006).
Sherer, D., and M. Karinch. *Dr. David Sherer's Hospital Survival Guide: 100+ Ways to Make Your Hospital Stay Safe and Comfortable* (Washington: Adler and Robin, 2003).
Smith, P.B., M.M. Kenan, and M.E. Kunik. *Alzheimer's for Dummies* (Hoboken: Wiley, 2004).

Woodson, Cheryl E. *To Survive Caregiving.* West Conshohocken, PA: Infinity, 2007.

Worden, J.W. *Grief Counseling and Grief Therapy.* New York: Springer Publishing, 2002.

Support Groups

American Red Cross
www.redcross.org/

Children of Aging Parents (CAPS)
P.O. Box 167
Richboro, PA 18954
1-800-227-7294
www.caps4caregivers.org

Family Caregiver Alliance
180 Montgomery St, Suite 1100
San Francisco, CA 94104
1-415-434-3388 or 1-800-445-8106
www.caregiver.org

Family Caregiving 101
www.familycaregiving101.org

National Academy of Elder Law Attorneys
www.naela.com

National Alliance for Caregiving
4720 Montgomery Lane, 2nd Floor
Bethesda, MD 20814
www.caregiving.org

National Association of Professional Geriatric Care Managers, Inc.
1-520-881-8808
www.caremanager.org

National Family Caregiver Support Program
http://www.agingcarefl.org/caregiver/NationalSupport

National Family Caregivers Association
10400 Connecticut Ave., #500
Kensington, MD 20895-3944
1-800-896-3650
www.nfcacares.org

SeniorBridge
1-866-506-1212
www.seniorbridge.com

Well Spouse Association
63 W Main Street, Suite H
Freehold, NJ 07728
1-800-838-0879
www.wellspouse.org

Government-Sponsored Medical and Health Websites

Administration of Aging, Eldercare Locator
Department of Health and Human Services
Washington, DC 20201
1-800-677-1116
www.aoa.gov

Food and Drug Administration
1-888-INFO-FDA
www.fda.gov

HealthFinder, sponsored by the U.S. Department of Health and Human Services
www.healthfinder.gov

Medline Plus, sponsored by the U.S. National Library of Medicine (NLM) and the National Institutes of Health (NIH)
www.medlineplus.gov

National Center for Complementary and Alternative Medicine
www.nccam.nih.gov

National Institute on Aging Information Center
1-800-222-4225
1-301-496-1752
www.niapublications.org

National Institutes of Health Senior Health
www.nihseniorhealth.gov

Disease-Specific Organizations and Websites

Alzheimer's Association
225 North Michigan Ave., Floor 17
Chicago, IL 60601
1-800-272-3900
www.alz.org

American Cancer Society
1-800-ACS-2345
www.cancer.org

American Chronic Pain Foundation
http://www.theacpa.org

American Heart Association
7272 Greenville Ave.
Dallas, TX 75231
1-800-AHA-USA1
www.heart.org/HEARTORG

Arthritis Foundation
P.O. Box 7669
Atlanta, GA 30357-0669
1-800-283-7800
www.arthritis.org

National Osteoporosis Foundation
1-800-231-4222
www.nof.org

National Parkinson Foundation
1501 NW 9th Ave./Bob Hope Road
Miami, FL 33136-1494
1-800-473-4636
www.parkinson.org

Medical Organizations

American Academy of Orthopaedic Surgeons
www.orthoinfo.org

American Association of Family Physicians (AAFP)
www.familydoctor.org

American Board of Medical Specialties
www.abms.org

American Medical Association
www.ama-assn.org

American College of Physicians, Internal Medicine
www.acponline.org/patients_families/

American College of Rheumatology
www.rheumatology.org

American College of Surgeons
www.facs.org

Internet References

AARP. "How to Deal with Long-Distance Issues." http://www.aarp.org/relationships/caregiving-resource-center/info-09-2010/pc_tips_for_long_distance_caregiver.html.
Adams, C.P., and V.V. Brantner. "Estimating the Cost of New Drug Development: Is It Really $802 Million?" *Health Affairs* 25, no.2 (2006): 420–428. http://content.healthaffairs.org/cgi/content/full/25/2/420.
Administration on Aging. "Heat Illnesses and Tips for Preventing Illness During Hot Weather." http://www.aoa.gov/AoARoot/Preparedness/Resources_Individuals/Heat_Illness.aspx.
AGS Foundation for Health in Aging. "Preventing Serious Falls: Tips for Older Adults and Their Loved Ones." http://www.healthinaging.org/public_education/falls_tips.pdf.
Alzheimer's Association. "Brain Tour." http://www.alz.org/alzheimers_disease_4719.asp.
Alzheimer's Association, "Dressing and Grooming," http://alz.org/living_with_alzheimers_dressing_and_grooming.asp.
Alzheimer's Association. "Standard Treatments." http://www.alz.org/alzheimers_disease_standard_prescriptions.asp.

Alzheimer's Association. "10 Warning Signs of Alzheimer's Disease." http://www.alz.org/alzheimers_disease_10_signs_of_alzheimers.asp.

Alzheimer's Association. "What Is Alzheimers?" http://www.alz.org/alzheimers_disease_what_is_alzheimers.asp.

Alzheimer's Research Foundation. "10 Tips for Traveling with Your Loved One," http://www.alzinfo.org/06/articles/caregiving-52.

Alzheimer's Society. "Mediterranean Diet Decreases Dementia." International Conference on Alzheimer's Disease, 2009. http://www.alzheimers.org.uk/site/scripts/news_article.php?newsID=506.

American Academy of Family Doctor. "Antibiotics: When They Can and Can't Help." http://familydoctor.org/online/famdocen/home/common/infections/protect/680.html.

American Academy of Orthopaedic Surgeons (AAOS), "Viscosupplement Treatment for Arthritis," http://www.orthoinfo.asos.org/topic.cfm?topic=a00217.

American Cancer Society. Cancer Facts and Figures, 2010. http://www.cancer.org/acs/groups/content/@epidemiologysurveilance/documents/document/acsp.c-026238.pdf.

American Cancer Society. "Diet and Physical Activity: What's the Cancer Connection?" http://www.cancer.org/Cancer/CancerCauses/DietandPhysicalActivity/diet-and-physical-activity.

American Cancer Society. "Guidelines for the Early Detection of Cancer." http://www.cancer.org/Healthy/FindCancerEarly/CancerScreeningGuidelines/american-cancer-society-guidelines-for-the-early-detection-of-cancer.

American Cancer Society. "How Do I Protect Myself from UV?" http://www.cancer.org/Cancer/CancerCauses/SunandUVExposure/SkinCancerPreventionandEarlyDetection/skin-cancer-prevention-and-early-detection-u-v-protection.

American Cancer Society. "Signs and Symptoms of Cancer." http://www.cancer.org/Cancer/CancerBasics/signs-and-symptoms-of-cancer.

American Cancer Society. "What in Cigarette Smoke Is Harmful?" http://www.cancer.org/Cancer/CancerCauses/TobaccoCancer/QuestionsaboutSmokingTobaccoandHealth/questions-about-smoking-tobacco-and-health-cancer-and-health.

American Dental Association. "Preventing Periodontal Disease." *Journal of American Dental Association* 132 (September 2001). http://www.ada.org/sectdions/ScienceAndResearch/pdfs/patient_08.pdf.

American Diabetes Association. "Checking Your Blood Glucose." http://www.diabetes.org/living-with-diabetes/treatment-and-care/blood-glucose-control/checking-your-blood-glucose.html.

American Diabetes Association. "Diet, Exercise, Anti-diabetic Drugs Can Delay or Prevent Type 2 Diabetes for 10+ Years." http://www.diabetes.org/news-research/research/recent/recent-advances/diet-exercise-anti-….

American Geriatrics Society, Foundation for Health in Aging. "Avoid Overmedication and Harmful Drug Reactions." http://www.healthinaging.org/public_education/avoiding_overmedication.pdf.

American Geriatrics Society, Foundation for Health in Aging. "Emergency Preparedness Tips for Older Adults." http://www.healthinaging.org/public_education/emergency_tips.php.

American Geriatrics Society, Foundation for Health in Aging. "Winter Safety Tips for Older Adults." http://www.healthinaging.org/public_education/wintersafety_tips.pdf.

American Heart Association. "Abnormal Cholesterol Levels May Raise Risk of Heart Attack." http://newsroom.heart.org/pr/aha/898.aspx.

American Heart Association, "Heart Disease and Stroke Statistics—2011 Update," http://circ.ahajournals.org/content/123/4/e18.full.pdf.

American Heart Association. "More Hospitals Administering Emergency Stroke Drug, but Many Patients Don't Seek Treatment Quickly Enough to Get It." http://www.newsroom.heart.org/pr/aha/833.aspx.

American Heart Association (AHA). "Reality Check." http://americanheart.biz/HEARTORG/Caregiver/RealityCheck/RealityCheckIntroduction/Reality-Check-Introduction_UCM_301769_Article.jsp.

American Heart Association. "Rejuvenate." http://www.heart.org/HEARTORG/Caregiver/Rejuvenate/RejuvenateIntroduction/Rejuvenate-Introduction_UCM_301816_Article.jsp.

American Heart Association. "Smoking and Cardiovascular Disease." http://www.heart.org/HEARTORG/GettingHealthy/QuitSmoking/QuittingResources/Smoking-Cardiovascular-Disease_UCM_305187_Article.jsp.

American Heart Association. "Smoking Remains Potent Risk Factor for Death from Heart Disease, Cancer." http://www.newsroom.heart.org/pr/aha/897.aspx.

American Heart Association. "Why Blood Pressure Matters." http://www.heart.org/HEARTORG/Conditions/HighBloodPressure/WhyBloodPressureMatters/Why-Blood-Pressure-Matters_UCM_002051_Article.jsp.

American Heart Association. "Women and Cardiovascular Diseases, 2011 Update," http://heart.org/idc/groups/heart-public/@wcm/@sop/@smd/documents/downloadable/ucm_319576.pdf.

American Massage Therapy Association (AMTA). "Massage and Serious Health Conditions." http://www.amtamassage.org/findamassage/health_conditions.html.

American Massage Therapy Association (AMTA). "Massage Therapy Can Relieve Stress." http://www.amtamassage.org/statement2.html.

American Occupational Therapy Association Fact Sheet. "Home Modifications and Occupational Therapy." http://www.aota.org/Practitioners/PracticeAreas/Rehab/Tools/38511.aspx.

American Sleep Apnea Association. *Tired of the Sleepiness?* http://www.sleepapnea.org/resources/brochure.html.

American Sleep Apnea Association. "Treatment Options for Adults with Obstructive Sleep Apnea." http://www.sleepapnea.org/resources/pubs/treatment.html.

American Stroke Association, "Warning Signs," http://www.strokeassociation.org/STROKEORG/Warning Signs/Warning_Signs_UCM_308528_SUBHOMEPAGE.jsp.

Area Agency on Aging of Pasco-Pinellas. "Are You a Caregiver?" http://www.agingcarefl.org/caregiver/caregiver.

Arthritis Foundation. Osteoarthritis Fact Sheet. http://www.arthritis.org/media/newsroom/osteoarthritis_Fact_Sheet_from_AF-Find_12_10_09.pdf.

Ata, Ashar, J. Lee, S. Bestle, J. Desemone, and S. Stain. "Postoperative Hyperglycemia and Surgical Site Infection in General Surgery Patients." *Archives of Surgery* 145, no. 9 (September 2010). http://archsurg.ama-assn.org/cgi/content/short/145/9/858.

ATMA. "Choosing a Type of Massage." www.amtamassage.org/findamassage/massage_type.html.

Austin, L. "Children as Caregivers." *Today's Caregiver.* http://www.caregiver.com/articles/children/children_as_caregivers.htm.

Berent, R., J. Auer, P. Schmid, G. Krannmair, S.F. Crouse, and J.S. Green. "Periodontal and Coronary Heart Disease in Patients Undering Coronary Angiography." *Metabolism* 60, no, 1 (2011): 127–133. http://www.ncbi.nlm.nih.gov/pubmed/20096894.

Caregiver Resource Center. Corporate Services. http://www.caregiverresourcecenter.com/corporate_services.htm.

Caregivers Library. "Infection Control." http://www.caregiverslibrary.org/Default.aspx?tabid=481.

CBS News. "Bad Habits Can Age You by 12 Years, Study Shows." http://www.cbsnews.com/stories/2010/04/26/health/main6434223.shtml.

CDC. "Falls Among Older Adults: An Overview." http://www.cdc.gov/HomeandRecreationalSafety/Falls/adultfalls.html.

Census Reports. "Twelfth Census of the United States Taken in Year 1900." http://www.cdc.gov/nchs/data/vsushistorical/vsush_1900_3.pdf.

Center for the Advancement of Health. "Depression Alters Immune Systems by Depressing Physical Activity." *ScienceDaily* (November 20, 1999). http://www.sciencedaily.com/releases/1999/11/991130062958.htm.

Centers for Disease Control. "Be Healthy and Safe in the Garden." http://cdc.gov/features/gardeningtips.

Centers for Disease Control (CDC). "Deaths: Final Data for 2005." http://www.cdc.gov/nchs/data/nvsr/nvsr56/nvsr56_10.pdf.

Centers for Disease Control. "Health Benefits of Pets." http://www.cdc.gov/healthypets/health_benefits.htm.

Centers for Disease Control (CDC). National Diabetes Fact Sheet, 2007. http://www.cdc.gov/diabetes/pubs/pdf/ndfs_2007.pdf.

Centers for Disease Control (CDC). "Ten Great Public Health Achievements — United States, 1900–1999." http://cdc.gov/mmwr/preview/mmwrhtml/00056796.htm.

Centers for Disease Control and Prevention (CDC). "Wash Your Hands." http://www.cdc.gov/Features/HandWashing/.

Centers for Medicare and Medicaid. "Medicare and You." http://www.medicare.gov/Publications/Pubs/pdf/10050.pdf.

Centers for Medicare and Medicaid Services. "Medicare Hospice Benefits," http://www.medicare.gov/Publications/Pubs/pdf/02154.pdf.

Children of Aging Parents. "Strategies for Avoiding Burnout During Caregiving." http://www.caps4caregivers.org/Assets/CAPSsummer2007B.pdf.

Childstats.gov. "America's Children: Key National Indicators of Well-being, 2009 Highlights." http://childstats.gov/pdf/ac2009/ac_09.pdf.

Development for Professional Employees. "Professional Women: Vital Statistics Fact Sheet, 2006." http://www.pay-equity.org/PDFs/ProfWomen.pdf.

Diabetes Research Institute. "Under the Microscope: Interview with Norma S. Kenyon, Ph.D." http://ww.diabetesresearch.org/Page.aspx?pid=1134.

Family Caregiver Alliance. Fact Sheet. "Taking Care of YOU: Self-Care for Family Caregivers." http://www.caregiver.org/caregiver/jsp/content_node.jsp?nodeid=847.

Family Caregiver Alliance. "Siblings and Caregiving." http://www.caregiver.org/caregiver/jsp/content_node.jsp?nodeid=653.

Family Caregivers Online. Module 9. "Caring for the Caregiver." www.familycaregiversonline.com/family_caregiver_module.asp?module=17.

Family Doctor.org. "Tips for Talking to Your Doctor." http://familydoctor.org/online/famdocen/home/pat-advocacy/healthcare/837.html.

"Fight-or-Flight Versus Tend-and-Befriend: The Significance of Gender Differences in Stress Responses." http://obssr.od.nih.gov/pdf/taylor_slides.pdf.

Freedom from Fear. "An Overview of Depression." http://www.freedomfromfear.org/depressionoverview.asp.

Gallup News Service. "Very Religious Americans Lead Healthier Lives." December 23, 2010. http://www.gallup.com/poll/145379/Religious-Americans-Lead-Healthier-Lives.aspx.

Gallup News Service. "Who Believes in God and Who Doesn't?" June 23, 2006. http://www.gallup.com/poll/23470/Who-Believes-God-Who-Doesnt.aspx.

Hall, C.B., R.B. Lipton, M. Sliwinski, M.J. Katz, C.A. Derby, and J. Verghes. "Cognitive Activities Delay Onset of Memory Decline in Persons Who Develop Dementia." *Neurology* 73 (2009): 356–361. http://www.neurology.org/cgi/content/abstract/73/5/356.

Harvard School of Public Health. Press release. "Active Social Life May Delay Memory Loss Among U.S. Elderly Population." http://www.hsph.harvard.edu/news/press-releases/2008-releases/active-social-life-delay-memory-loss-us-elderly.html.

Health and Age. "Exercise Helps Caregivers Manage Stress." http://www.healthandage.org/Exercise-Aids-Stressed_Caregivers.

Health Journeys. "What Is Guided Imagery?" www.healthjourneys.com/what_is_guided_imagery.asp.

Heart Rhythm Society. "INR." http://www.heartrhythmfoundation.org/a-fib/INR_FINAL.pdf.

Holistic Online. "Therapeutic Benefits of Laughter." http://www.holisticonline.com/Humor_Therapy/humor_therapy_benefits.htm.

Hypography Science for Everyone, "High Heels Bad News for Knees," http://hypography.com/news/life-sciences/30688.html.

Intelihealth. "Meditation." http://www.intelihealth.com/IH/ihtIH?d=dmtContent&c=362173&p=~br,IHW~st,24479~r,WSIHW000x~b,*.

InterNACHI. "Home Safety for the Elderly." http://www.nachi.org/elderlysafety.hml.

International Conference on Alzheimer's Disease (ICAD). 2009 press release. http://www.alzheimers.org.uk/site/scripts/news_article.php?newsID=499.

The Joint Commission. Speak UP Initiative. "Five Things You Can Do to Prevent Infection." http://www.jointcommission.org/Speak_Up_Five_Things_You_Can_Do_To_Prevent_Infection/.

King's College. "Exercise in Leisure Time Prolongs Life." http://www.kcl.ac.uk/news/news_details.php?year=2008&news_id=729.

Kubler-Ross, Elisabeth, and David Kessler. "The Five Stages of Grief." http://grief.com/the-five-stages-of-grief/.

Kvaavik, E., D. Batty, G. Ursin, R. Huxley, and C. Gale. "Influence of Individual and Combined Health Behaviors on Total and Cause-Specific Mortality in Men and Women." *Archives of Internal Medicine* 170, no. 8. http://archinte.ama-assn.org/cgi/content/short/170/8/711.

Mayo Clinic. "Diabetes and Alzheimer's Linked." http://www.mayoclinic/health/diabetes-and-alzheimers/AZ00050/.

MayoClinic.com. "Forgiveness: How to Let Go of Grudges and Bitterness." http://www.mayoclinic.com/health/forgiveness/MH00131/.

MayoClinic.com. "Healthy Lifestyles." http://www.mayoclinic.com/health/HealthyLivingIndex/HealthyLivingIndex.

Medical News Today, "Staying Lean and Fit Reduced Men's Risk of Heart Failure," http://medicalnewstoday.com/articles/134128.php.

Medicare.gov. Medicare Advantage Part C. http://www.medicare.gov/navigation/medicare-basics/medicare-benefits/part-c.aspx.

Medline Plus. "Partial Thromboplastin Time (PTT)." http://www.nlm.nih.gov/medlineplus/ency/article/003653.htm.

Medline Plus. "Prothrombin Time (PT)." http://www.nlm.nih.gov/medlineplus/ency/article/003652.htm.

National Alliance for Caregiving. "Young Caregivers in the U.S." http://www.caregiving.org/data/youngcaregivers.pdf.

National Center for Complementary and Alternative Medicine (NCCAM). "Acupuncture Relieves Pain and Improves Function in Knee Osteoarthritis." http://nccam.nih.gov/research/results/spotlight/052504.htm.

National Center for Complementary and Alternative Medicine, National Institutes of Health. National Institutes of Health news advisory. "More than One-Third of U.S. Adults Use Complementary and Alternative Medicine, According to New Government Survey." http://nccam.nih.gov/news/2004/052704.htm.

National Center for Health Statistics. "Overweight Prevalence Among Adults, 2005–2006." http://www.cdc.gov/nchs/data/hestat/overweight/overweight_adult.htm.

National Family Caregiver. "Caregivers and Your Health: How to Manage Stress." http://nfcacares.org/pdfs/Evercare_caregiver_stress.pdf.

National Family Caregivers Association. "The Best Present You Can Give Your Loved One: Your Own Good Health." http://www.nfcacares.org/pdfs/ProtectYourHealth.pdf.

National Family Caregivers Association. Caregiving Statistics. http://www.nfcacares.org/who_are_family_caregivers/care_giving_statstics.cfm.

National Family Caregivers Association. "The Stress of Family Caregiving." http://nfcacares.org/pdfs/TakeCareWinter06.pdf.

National Family Caregivers Association. "21st Century Caregiving—Then and Now." http://www.thefamilycaregiver.org/who_are_family_caregivers/then_and_now.cfm.

National Heart, Lung and Blood Institute. *Your Guide to Lowering Blood Pressure.* http://www.nhlbi.nih.gov/health/public/heart/hbp/hbp_low/hbp_low.pdf.

National Institute of Arthritis and Musculoskeletal and Skin Diseases. "Osteoarthritis." http://www.niams.nih.gov/Health_Info/Osteoarthritis/default.asp#2.

National Institute of Diabetes and Digestive and Kidney Diseases, National Institutes of Health (NIH). "DCCT and EDIC: The Diabetes Control and Complications Trial and Follow-up Study." http://diabetes.niddk.nih.gov/dm/pubs/control/index.htm.

National Institute of Mental Health. "Research Shows How Chronic Stress May Be Linked to Physical and Mental Ailments." http://www.nimh.nih.gov/science-news/2009/research-shows-how-chronic-stress-may-be-linked-to-physical-and-mental-ailments.shtml.

National Institute of Neurological Disorders. "Brain Basics: Understanding Sleep." http://www.ninds.nih.gov/disorders/brain_basics/understanding_sleep.htm.

National Institutes of Health. "Alzheimer's Disease Genetics Fact Sheet." http://www.nia.nih.gov/Alzheimers/Publications/geneticsfs.htm.

National Institutes of Health. "Can Pets Help Keep You Healthy?" http://newsinhealth.nih.gov/2009/February/feature1.htm.

National Institutes of Health. "Sleep Apnea Tied to Increased Risk of Stroke." http://www.nih.gov/news/health/apr2010/nhlbi-08.htm.

National Institutes of Health (NIH). "Stressed Out?" http://newsinhealth.nih.gov/pdf/NIHNiHJanuary07.pdf.

National Sleep Foundation. "Can't Sleep? What to Know About Insomnia." http://www.sleepfoundation.org/article/sleep-related-problems/insomnia-and-sleep.

National Sleep Foundation. "One-Third of Americans Lose Sleep over Economy." http://www.sleepfoundation.org/article/press-release/one-third-americans-lose-sleep-over-economy.

National Stroke Foundation. "Warning Signs of Stroke." http://www.stroke.org/site/PageNavigator/ALS_Splash_20110907.html.

NCCAM. "Dietary Supplements Glucosamine and/or Chondroitin Fare No Better than Placebo in Slowing Structural Damage of Knee Osteoarthritis." http://nccam.nih.gov/news/2008/092908.htm.

Nurses Health Study. *The Nurses' Health Study Annual Newsletter* 14 (2007). http://www.channing.harvard.edu/nhs/wp-content/uploads/n2007.pdf.

"Prayer and Spirituality in Health: Ancient Practices, Modern Science." www.jpsych.com/pdfs/NCCAM-PrayerandSpirituality.pdf

"Precise Neurological Exam." http://edinfo.med.nyu.edu/courseware/neurosurgery/sensory.html.

Ramos, M. Mindmovers. "Music Therapy." http://www.mindmovers.com/store/music.htm.

Rand Corporation. "Why People Overeat." http://www.rand.org/pubs/research_briefs/RB9327/index1.html.

Research in Review. "A Book for the Mind." http://www.rinr.fsu.edu/fallwinter9899/features/book.html.

Robiner, W. "Psychological and Physical Reactions to Whirlpool Baths." *Journal of Behavioral Medicine* 13, no. 2 (1900): 157–173. http://www.springerlink.com/content/r100363044650082/.

Rubenstein, Laurence Z. "Falls in Older People: Epidemiology, Risk Factors and Strategies for Prevention." *Age and Ageing* (2006): 35–52. http://ageing.oxfordjournals.org/content/35/suppl_2/ii37.full.pdf.

Science Daily. "Comfort-food Cravings May Be Body's Attempt to Put Brake on Chronic Stress." http://www.sciencedaily.com/releases/2003/09/030911072109.htm.

Tonetti, M.S., F. D'Aiuto, L. Nibali, A. Donald, C. Storrey, M. Parkar, J. Suvan, A. Hingorani, P. Vallance, and J. Deanfield. "Treatment of Periodontitis and Endothelial Function." *New England Journal of Medicine* 356: 911–920. http://www.nejm.org/doi/full/10.1056/NEJMoa063186.

U.S. Department of Health and Human Services, Administration of Aging. "Be Wise … Immunize." http://www.caregiver.org/caregiver/jsp/content/pdfs/English_final 1.2.pdf.

U.S. Department of Health and Human Services, Centers for Disease Control and Prevention. National Health Statistics Reports, July 30, 2008. http://www.cdc.gov/nchs/data/nhsr/nhsr005.pdf.

U.S. Department of Health and Human Services. "Health, United States, 2007." www.cdc.gov/nchs/data/hus/hus07.pdf#027.

U.S. Department of Health and Human Services, National Diabetes Education Program. "The Facts About Diabetes: America's Seventh Leading Cause of Death." http://ndep.nih.gov/diabetes-facts/index.aspx.

U.S. Department of Health and Human Services, National Diabetes Education Program. "Small Steps, Big Rewards: Your GAME PLAN to Prevent Type 2 Diabetes." Information for Patients. http://ndep.nih.gov/publications/PublicationDetail.aspx?PubId=71.

U.S. Department of Health and Human Services, NIH National Diabetes Education Program. "Get Real! You Don't Have to Knock Yourself Out to Prevent Diabetes." http://ndep.nih.gov/publications/PublicationDetail.aspx?PubId=76.

U.S. Department of Health and Human Services. "A Statistical Profile of Older Americans Aged 65+." www.h-gac.com/human-services/aging/documents/AStatisticalProfileofOlderAmericansAged65plus.pdf.

U.S. Department of Labor, Employment Standards Administration. Family and Medical Leave Act. http://www.dol.gov/whd/fmla/finalrule/factsheet.pdf.

University of Chicago. "Polypharmacy in Older Adults." http://prescriptions.uchicago.edu/Polypharmacy/symptoms.html.

University of Iowa Health Science Relations. "Children and Critically Ill Parents: What Children Need to Know." http://www.uihealthcare.com/topics/medicaldepartments/pediatrics/childrenillparents/index.html.

University of Pennsylvania School of Medicine. "Targeting Tau: Inflammation Study

Suggests New Approach for Fighting Alzheimer's." http://www.uphs.upenn.edu/news/News_Releases/jan07/microglia-activation-alzheimers.htm.
USAA Education Foundation. "Effects of Aging on Driving Skills." www.usaaedfoundation.org/DownloadRelatedForm/535_Recent_Driving_Experiences_Checklist.pdf.
WebMD. "Caregiver Burnout." http://women.webmd.com/caregiver-recognizing-burnout.
WebMD. "Caregivers Tip No. 1: Take Care of Yourself First." http://www.webmd.com/balance/tc/caregiver-tips-caregiver-tip-number-1-take-care-of-yourself-first.
WebMD. "Frostbite Treatment." http://firstaid.webmd.com/frostbite-treatment.
WebMD. "Understanding Heat-Related Illness — Treatment." http://firstaid.webmd.com/understanding-heat-related-illness-treatment.
WebMD.com. "His and Hers Stress Advice." http://women.webmd.com/features/stress-tips-for-men-and-women/.
Wilson, R.S., K.R. Krueger, S.E. Arnold, SE, J.A. Schneider, J.F. Kelly, L.L. Barnes et al. "Loneliness and Risk of Alzheimer's Disease." *Archives of General Psychiatry* 64, no. 2 (2007): 234–240. http://archpsyc.ama-assn.org/cgi/content/abstract/64/2/234.
Zimney, E. "Gardening Is Good Exercise." http://www.everydayhealth.com/blog/zimney-health-and-medical-news-you-can-use/gardening-is-good-exercise/.

Evaluating Web-Based Health Resources

SOURCE: National Center for Complementary and Alternative Medicine (NCCAM), Evaluating Web-Based Health Resources, http://www.nccam.nih.gov/health/webresources/

Who runs the site? Any reliable health-related Web site should make it easy for you to learn who is responsible for the site and its information. On the National Institutes of Health (NIH) Web site, for example, each major page clearly identifies NIH and includes a link to the site's homepage. The National Center for Complementary and Alternative Medicine (NCCAM) Web site follows the same practice; because NCCAM is part of NIH, the NCCAM site's major pages also link to the NIH homepage.

Who pays for the site? It costs money to run a Web site. The source of a Web site's funding should be clearly stated or readily apparent. For example, Web addresses (such as NCCAM's) ending in ".gov" denote a government-sponsored site; ".edu" indicates an educational institution, ".org" a noncommercial organization, and ".com" a commercial organization. You should know how the site pays for its existence. Does it sell advertising? Is it sponsored by a drug company? The source of funding can affect what content is presented, how the content is presented, and what the site owners want to accomplish on the site. (For example, if a site about osteoarthritis is funded by a manufacturer of a drug or dietary supplement that people might use for this condition, that could affect the site's content.) If the funding source is unclear, or if it is a person or an organization with a proprietary interest in the information presented, try to confirm the information elsewhere (e.g., studies published in scientific journals, or government-sponsored Web sites).

Purpose of the Site. The site's purpose is related to who runs and pays for it. Look for an "About this site" link on the home page. There you should find a clear statement of purpose, which will help you evaluate the trustworthiness of the information.

Information Sources. Many health/medical sites post information collected from other Web sites or sources. If the person or organization in charge of the site did not create the information, the original source should be clearly labeled.

Basis of the Information. In addition to identifying who wrote the material you are reading, the site should describe the evidence (such as articles in medical journals) that the material is based on. Also, opinions or advice should be clearly set apart from information that is "evidence-based" that is, based on research results. For example, if a site discusses health benefits people can expect from treatment, look for references to scientific research that clearly supports what is said. Keep in mind that testimonials, anecdotes, unsupported claims, and opinions are not the same as objective, evidence-based information. Remember: if something sounds too good to be true, it probably is.

How the Information Is Selected and Reviewed. If a Web site is presenting medical information, people with credible professional and scientific qualifications should review the material before it is posted. Check for the presence of an editorial board, or other indications of how information is selected and reviewed.

Whether the Information Is Current. Web sites should be reviewed and updated on a regular basis. It is particularly important that medical information be current — outdated content can be midleading or even dangerous. The most recent update or review date should be clearly posted. (For example, this information appears at the end of all of the fact sheets posted on NCCAM's Web site.) Even if the information has not changed, you want to know whether the site ownders have reviewed it recently to ensure that it is still valid.

Links to Other Sites. Web sites usually have a policy about establishing links to other sites. Some medical sites take a conservative approach and don't link to any other sites. Some link to any site that asks, or pays, for a link. Others only link to sites that have met certain criteria.

Personal Information. Web sites routinely track visitors' paths to determine what pages are being viewed. A health Web site may ask you to "subscribe" or "become a member." In some cases, this may be so that it can collect a user fee or select information for you that is relevant to your concerns. In all cases, this will give the site personal information about you.

Any credible site asking for this kind of information should tell you exactly what it will and will not do with it. Many commercial sites sell "aggregate" (collected) data about their users to other companies — information such as what percentage of their users are women older than 40, for example. In some cases, they may collect and reuse information that is "personally identifiable," such as your ZIP code, gender, and birth date. Be sure to read any privacy policy or similar language on the site, and don't sign up for anything you don't fully understand.

Interacting with a Site. You should always be able to contact the site owner if you run across problems or have questions or feedback. If the site hosts chat rooms or other online discussion areas, it should explain the terms of using this service. Is it moderated? If so, by whom and why? Spend some time reading the discussion before joining in, to see whether you feel comfortable with the environment.

This fact sheet was adapted from the National Cancer Institute publication "Evaluating Health Information on the Internet," available at the NCI Web site at www.cancer.gov/cancertopics/factsheet/information/internet.

Additional resources include the following:

"Evaluating Health Web Sites," National Network of Libraries of Medicine, http://nnlm.gov/outreach/consumer/evalsite.html.

"Evaluating Internet Health Information: A Tutorial from the National Library of Medicine," http://www.nlm.nih.gov/medlineplus/webeval/webeval.html.

MedlinePlus Guide to Health Web Surfing," National Library of Medicine and National Institutes of Health, http://www.nlm.nih.gov/medlineplus/healthywebsurfing.html.

Index

AARP *see* American Association of Retired Persons
A1C (glycated hemoglobin test for diabetes) 208, 213, 216, 217
Abel, Emily 60
acceptance (final stage of grief) 22, 23, 55, 144
activities of daily living (ADL) 79, 130, 174, 183
advanced practice nurses (APN) or nurse practitioner 78
aerobic exercise 55, 184, 234
agency of aging 16, 131
Alzheimer, Dr. Alois 71
Alzheimer's Association 42, 72, 80, 168, 169, 171, 173, 175
Alzheimer's Disease 13, 38, 41, 72, 85, 162, 165–178
American Academy of Family Physicians 77, 88
American Association of Retired Persons (AARP) 15, 43, 47
American Bar Association 127, 140
American Board of Medical Specialty 76
American Cancer Society (ACS) 35, 39, 195, 196, 202, 203, 204, 205
American College of Surgeons 76, 77
American Geriatrics Society 87, 132, 135, 139
American Heart Association 32, 34, 36, 39, 41, 80, 153, 156, 223–235

American Massage Therapy Association 52, 189
American Medical Association (AMA) 76
American Red Cross 71
anesthesiology 67
anger (2nd stage of grief) 22, 55
angiogram and balloon angioplasty 226
anticipatory grief 146, 147
Arthritis Foundation 49, 155, 179, 180, 183, 187, 191, 192
The Arthritis Helpbook 183
articular cartilage 179, 181
atherosclerosis 158, 162, 225
Auguste, D, Frau 71, 72
Aviv, Abraham 154

Bacon, Roger 68
bargaining (3rd stage of grief) 22, 55
Barton, Clara 70, 71
Bennett, C. Kip 193, 199, 206
Bennett, Eric 193, 199, 206
Bickerdyke, Mary "Mother" 71
blood lipid panel (cholesterol, triglycerides, HDL, LDL) 50, 157, 158, 219, 225, 232, 234
blood pressure 157, 161, 166, 172, 188, 189, 190, 215, 217, 219, 228, 231, 232
board certified doctor 76, 77
Bond, Katie 207, 213
bone scan 197
Boylston, Dr Zabdiel (and small pox inoculation) 62, 63

269

brachytherapy 200
brand name drugs 89
Brotherton, Abigail 21, 22, 23, 24, 25, 26
Brotherton, Ashley 21, 22, 23, 24, 25, 26
Brotherton, Cindy 21, 22, 23, 24, 25, 26
Brotherton, Jerry 21, 22, 23, 24, 25, 26
Brotherton, Lindsey 21, 22, 23, 24, 25, 26

cancer 6, 22, 34, 35, 38, 41, 52, 72, 73, 74, 75, 80, 82, 85, 86, 87, 88, 94, 117, 147, 164, 193–206, 224, 225, 230, 232, 233
cardiac catherization 226
cardiovascular disease 34, 161, 221, 224, 231, 233
caregiver burnout 38, 39
Caregiving (Beth McLeon) 16
caregiving: long-term 8; role reversal 91; short-term 8; stages 10
Centers for Disease Control (CDC) 56, 115, 121, 154
certified registered nurse anesthetists (CRNA) 67, 78, 82, 113
Chain, Ernst 69
chemistry-7 blood test 101
chemotherapy 73, 78, 104, 198, 199, 200, 201, 205
Cherkas, Dr Lynn 154
chest x-ray 117, 229
chondrocyte 181, 182
clotting time blood tests (Prothrombin time, INR, Partial Thromboplastin Time or PTT) 117, 118
Cognex 72
collagen 181
Colton, Gardner 66
complete blood count (CBC) 116, 117
congestive heart failure (CHF) 34, 141, 224, 228, 229, 234, 235
The Courage to Laugh 54
Crick, Francis 205
Crile, George W. 67
cryosurgery 199
CT scan 193, 197, 227, 229
Cushing, Harvey 67

Davy, Humphrey 66
deep breathing and relaxation exercises 21
De Humani Corporis Fabrica (On the Contruction of the Human Body) 73
De Motu Cordis (On the Motion of the Heart) 73

denial (1st stage of grief) 22, 55
depression (among caregivers) 9, 19, 22, 36, 37, 38, 39, 50, 52, 87, 113, 143, 148, 149, 175, 183, 235
depression (4th stage of grief) 22, 23, 55
diabetes mellitus, type 1 209, 207–224
diabetes mellitus, type 2 (non-insulin dependent diabetes) 207–224
dietitians and nutritionists 78
Dix, Dorothea 70
DNA (deoxyribose nucleic acid) 65, 154, 196, 200, 205
Dr. David Scherer's HOSPITAL Survival Guide 109
doctor of osteopathy (DO) 74
Dolly the cloned sheep 65
Down's syndrome 21, 25
durable power of attorney (POA) for health care 83, 102

electrocardiogram (EKG) 65, 67, 117, 225, 231
The Emotional Survival Guide for Caregivers 43

Family and Medical Leave Act of 1993 (FMLA) 17
Family Caregiver Alliance (FCA) 32, 45
Fleming, Sir Alexander 65, 68, 69
Florey, Howard 69
forgiveness 19, 20
Franklin, Benjamin 63
frostbite 137, 138

Galen 68, 72, 73
Galile, Galileo 68
gardening 52, 215
general surgery 75
generic drugs 89
geriatricians 171
Gile, Bob 46, 58, 68, 207, 221
Gile, Jan 46, 58, 68, 207, 221
glucagon 210, 211, 212
grief and grieving 22, 23, 24, 25, 28, 143, 144, 145, 146, 147, 148, 150, 151
Gross, Greg 141, 142, 147, 150
Gross, Keith 141, 142, 147, 150
Gross, Michael 141, 142, 147, 150
Gross, Peggy 141, 142, 147, 150
Gunn, Dr. John 61
Gunn's Domestic Medicine or Poor Man's Friend: In the Hours of Affliction, Pain and Sickness 61

Harvey, William 73
health insurance portability and accountability act (HIPAA) 83, 103
heart attack (myocardial infarction) 34, 225, 234
heart disease 6, 34, 40, 41, 51, 55, 81, 85, 86, 112, 153, 157, 161, 163, 164, 166, 195, 217, 223–235
Hearts of Wisdom, American Women Caring for Kin 60
heat exhaustion 135, 136
heat stroke 135, 136
Herrick, James 67
high blood pressure (hypertension) 9, 33, 86, 153, 155, 156, 157, 161, 166, 189, 217, 218, 228, 231, 232
Hill, Jessica 128
Hippocrates 67, 72, 73, 205
Hooke, Robert 68
hormone therapy (cancer treatment) 73, 201
hospice 8, 11, 12, 19, 20, 83, 84, 85, 127
hospitalist 82
humor 39, 42, 54, 55, 151
hydrotherapy 49
hyperosmolar hyperglycemic state (HHS) 219, 220
hypoglycemia 219, 220
hypothermia 136, 137

If Only I'd Had This Caregiving Book 176
immunotherapy 73, 201
inoculation (vaccinations) 35, 63, 91, 115
insomnia 38, 39, 40, 188
instrumental activities of daily living (IADL) 79, 130
insulin 35, 65, 152, 153, 167, 209, 210, 211, 212, 214, 215, 216, 219, 220, 221
International Association of Certified Home Inspectors (InterNACHI) 134

Jackson, Dennis 67
Jacobs, Dr. Barry 42, 58, 80
John Hopkins' Hospital 64
Joint Commission of Accreditation of Healthcare Organizations (JCAHO) 81, 90, 91, 93, 96, 115, 122
journaling 55

ketoacidosis (diabetic) 212, 219, 220
Koch, Robert 68

laparoscopic surgery 75, 110, 111, 121, 199
laser 110, 199

Leeuwenhoek, Antoni van 68
Lewis, Thomas 67
licensed practical nurse (LPN) 78
licensed vocational nurse (LVN) 78
life expectancy 6, 41, 62
Lippershy, Hans 68
Lister, Joseph 68, 69
living will 14, 83, 108
Long, Crawford W. 66

malignant neoplasm 194, 196
mammogram 35, 196, 197
massage 51, 52
Mather, Cotton 62, 63
Medicaid 76, 84, 85
medical alert system 11, 131, 132, 138, 177
Medicare 75, 76, 84, 208, 217
meditation, prayer and spiritual support 187, 188, 189, 190
Mellanby, Edward 65
mesenchymal stem cells 220
miochondria of cell 33, 152, 196
Morgagni, Giovanni 73
Morgan, Dr. John 63
Morris, Lucien 67
Morton, William T. 66
MRI (magnetic resonance imaging) 82, 108, 173, 182, 197, 226, 227, 229
mucous membrane 114, 115, 186, 228
music 49, 51, 55, 56
My Book of Memories 177

National Cancer Institute 80
National Family Caregivers Association 17, 35
neoplasm 194, 196
neurology 171
neurosurgery 75
Nightingale, Florence 71
nucleus of cell 195

occupational therapist (OT) 15, 79, 183
oncologist surgeon 75
oncology 75, 194, 198, 199
oral glucose tolerance test (OGTT) 213, 214
orthopaedic surgeon 75, 107, 109, 182, 191, 192
osteoarthritis (degenerative joint disease) 109, 179–192
osteophyte 179, 181, 182
Oz, Dr. Mehmet 167, 215

Pardee, Harold 67
Pasteur, Louis 62, 65, 68, 69

pathology 75, 82, 198
penicillium 69
periodontal disease (gingivitis) 112, 153, 161, 162, 163, 164
PET scan 197, 198
pet therapy 56
pharmacy 19, 62, 79, 89, 97, 158, 175, 216
physical therapist (PT) 78, 79, 81, 127, 183, 184
plaques (Alzheimer's disease) 171, 176
platelets (thrombocytes) 116, 117, 200, 201, 230
polypharmacy 79, 86, 87
power of attorney (POA) 11, 80, 83, 127, 128
pre-admission testing and teaching (PATT) 116
Priestly, Joseph 66
primary care doctor 74, 75, 80, 108, 171, 182, 214
progressive muscle relaxation 49
psychiatry 143, 171
pulmonology 75

radiology 75, 82, 194, 198
red blood cells (RBC or erythrocytes) 116, 212, 213, 230
registered nurse (RN) 67, 77, 78, 82, 113
respiratory therapist (RT) 78, 79, 127
rheumatology 53, 75, 182
robot in surgery 110, 111
Roentgen, Wilhelm Conrad 64
Roizen, Dr. Michael 167, 215
role reversal in caregiving 91
Rush, Dr. Benjamin 64

Safford, Mary 71
sleep apnea 160, 161
Snow, John 66
social worker 11, 16, 28, 29, 42, 79, 85, 121, 130, 183

Spector, Tim 154
stages of grief (denial, anger, bargaining, depression and acceptance) 23, 145
strengthening exercises 184
stroke, hemorrhagic or ischemic (cardiovascular accident) 15, 43, 166, 217, 228, 234, 235
sudden death 147, 148
Sword, Brian 67

tai chi chuan 50, 53, 181, 184, 190
tangles (Alzheimer's disease) 171, 176
targeted therapy for cancer 201, 202
Taylor, Dr. Shelley 37
triglycerides 157, 212, 232, 234
211 Network 128–131

United States Army Nurses Corps 70

Vesalius, Andreas 73
visualization and guided imagery 49, 57, 190

walking (as exercise) 50, 51
Warren, John Collins 66
Washington, George 63
Waters, Dr Ralph 67
Watson, James 205
Wessel, Jack 38, 207, 208, 210, 216
Wessel, Sue 38, 207, 208, 210, 216
White, Dr. Paul Dudley 65
white blood cells (WBC or leukocytes) 116, 195, 200, 230

x-ray (radiograph) 67, 82, 107, 114, 116, 163, 181, 182

yoga 49, 50, 53, 150, 187, 190
YOU and Your Aging Parents 127, 128, 140

www.ingramcontent.com/pod-product-compliance
Ingram Content Group UK Ltd.
Pitfield, Milton Keynes, MK11 3LW, UK
UKHW041930140426
5217IPUK00014B/398